D0205182

Gastric Cytoprotection

A Clinician's Guide

Gastric Cytoprotection

A Clinician's Guide

Edited by

DANIEL HOLLANDER, M.D.

Division of Gastroenterology
Department of Medicine
University of California–Irvine
Irvine, California

and

ANDRZEJ S. TARNAWSKI, M.D., D.Sc.

Veterans Administration Medical Center
Long Beach, California
and Division of Gastroenterology
Department of Medicine
University of California – Irvine
Irvine, California

PLENUM MEDICAL BOOK COMPANY •
NEW YORK AND LONDON

Library of Congress Cataloging in Publication Data

Gastric cytoprotection / edited by Daniel Hollander and Andrzej S. Tarnawski.
  p.   cm.
  Includes bibliographies and index.
  ISBN 0-306-43266-8
  1. Peptic ulcer — Etiology.2. Gastric mucosa. I. Hollander, Daniel. II. Tarnawski, Andrzej.
  [DNLM: 1. Gastric Mucosa — cytology. 2. Gastric Mucosa — physiology. 3. Intestinal Mucosa — cytology.4. Intestinal Mucosa — physiology. WI 302 G2545]
  RC821.G37   1989
  616.3′43071 — dc20
  DNLM/DLC   89-16101
  for Library of Congress   CIP

© 1989 Plenum Publishing Corporation
233 Spring Street, New York, N.Y. 10013

Plenum Medical Book Company is an imprint of Plenum Publishing Corporation

Printed in the United States of America

Contributors

Adrian Allen • Department of Physiological Sciences, Medical School, University of Newcastle upon Tyne, Newcastle upon Tyne NE2 4HH, England

Gregory L. Eastwood • Gastroenterology Division, University of Massachusetts Medical School, Worcester, Massachusetts 01605

Daniel Hollander • Division of Gastroenterology, Department of Medicine, University of California–Irvine, Irvine, California 92717

Andrew C. Hunter • Department of Physiological Sciences, Medical School, University of Newcastle upon Tyne, Newcastle upon Tyne NE2 4HH, England

Jan W. Konturek • Institute of Physiology, Academy of Medicine, 31–531 Krakow, Poland

Stanislaw J. Konturek • Institute of Physiology, Academy of Medicine, 31–531 Krakow, Poland

Anwar H. Mall • Department of Physiological Sciences, Medical School, University of Newcastle upon Tyne, Newcastle upon Tyne NE2 4HH, England

Peter J. Oates • Central Research Division, Pfizer Inc., Department of Metabolic Diseases, Groton, Connecticut 06340

James Penston • Ninewells Hospital, Dundee DD1 9SY, Scotland

Wynne D. W. Rees • Department of Gastroenterology, Hope Hospital, University of Manchester School of Medicine, Salford M6 8HD, England

André Robert • Drug Metabolism Research, The Upjohn Company, Kalamazoo, Michigan 49001

Christopher J. Shorrock • Department of Gastroenterology, Hope Hospital, University of Manchester School of Medicine, Salford M6 8HD, England

Jerzy Stachura • Department of Cell Pathology, University Medical School, 31-531 Krakow, Poland; and Division of Gastroenterology, University of California–Irvine, Irvine, California 92717

Sandor Szabo • Department of Pathology, Brigham & Women's Hospital, and Department of Pathology, Harvard Medical School, Boston, Massachusetts 02115

Andrzej Tarnawski • Veterans Administration Medical Center, Long Beach, California 90822; and Division of Gastroenterology, Department of Medicine, University of California–Irvine, Irvine, California 92717

Donald E. Wilson • Department of Medicine, State University of New York, Health Science Center at Brooklyn, Brooklyn, New York 11203

Kenneth G. Wormsley • Ninewells Hospital, Dundee DD1 9SY, Scotland

.

Preface

Gastric secretions contain hydrogen ions at a concentration that is more than one million times higher than their intracellular concentration. This phenomenal gradient as well as the demonstrated ability of gastric juice to digest tissues has motivated clinicians and investigators alike to emphasize acid secretion and acid ablation in studying the pathogenesis and therapy of peptic ulcer disease. Consequently, over the past 150 years, we have made considerable progress in understanding the mechanisms and regulation of acid secretion by the stomach. Not surprisingly, therapy for both peptic disease and mucosal injury has also been predominantly directed at either neutralizing acid or suppressing its production.

During the past 10 years, attention has been focused on factors other than acid in the genesis and therapy of ulcer disease. Work done worldwide demonstrated that acid hypersecretion is not a common event in peptic ulcer disease. Therefore, we began realizing that factors other than acid secretion may be important in the genesis of ulcer disease or in gastroduodenal mucosal damage. In addition, new physiological information has established that the gastroduodenal mucosa is normally protected by a complex series of events including mucus and bicarbonate secretion, cell renewal, surface mucosal restitution, and preservation of the microvasculature and mucosal proliferative zone.

Our increased understanding of how the gastroduodenal mucosa protects itself has given rise to a general concept referred to as cytoprotection or mucosal protection. Concepts of cytoprotection have greatly enlarged our overall perspective of peptic ulcer disease and mucosal injury and have also resulted in the development of new therapeutic approaches to these problems. The cytoprotective approach uses drugs, such as prostaglandins, sucralfate, bismuth compounds, antacids, and dietary essential fatty acids, which are precursors of prostaglandin synthesis.

The concepts of cytoprotection and its specific mechanisms have been published primarily in journals or books oriented toward the investigator. Yet this new information needs to be transmitted from the research literature to the clinical arena. Clinicians must begin to understand these new and exciting concepts in order to be able to offer their patients newer therapies in addition to acid inhibition.

This book attempts to bridge this gap. The authors summarize the present state of our knowledge, simplify its presentation, and point out the therapeutic implications of this evolving field. The volume should help elucidate these concepts for general internists and gastroenterologists alike and, it is hoped, begin to bridge the gap between the research laboratory and medical practice.

Many of the concepts presented here are still in an evolutionary state. The precise mechanisms of how the gastroduodenal mucosa protects itself are not known. Therefore, the reader will have to be tolerant of some lack of clear-cut explanations for many of the observations. In addition, it should be borne in mind that we are presenting still-evolving information—information that is still fresh off the laboratory bench, and about which consensus has yet to be reached in the medical community. Therefore, the authors presenting the work may not necessarily agree with each other on every detail or every explanation.

The authors of these chapters are some of the leading experts in cytoprotection research. They present their personal views of the latest developments in their areas of expertise. We thank them for their enthusiastic support and willingness to contribute to this clinician-oriented book.

We want to thank our administrative assistant, Ms. Nancy Pharo, for her continuous help, and also to thank the many individuals at Plenum Publishing Corporation for their help and encouragement.

Daniel Hollander
Andrzej Tarnawski

Irvine, California

Contents

Chapter 3

Pathomorphology of Gastric Mucosal Injury 33

Jerzy Stachura

Chapter 6

Bicarbonate Secretion and the Alkaline Microclimate   91

Christopher J. Shorrock and Wynne D. W. Rees

Chapter 7

Epithelial Cell Renewal   109

Gregory L. Eastwood

Chapter 8

Gastric Blood Flow and Mucosal Defense 125

Peter J. Oates

Part III. Cytoprotective Therapy

Chapter 9

Cytoprotective Therapy: Prostaglandins 169
Donald E. Wilson

Chapter 10

**The Role of Nutrient Essential Fatty Acids
in Gastric Mucosal Protection** 187
Daniel Hollander and Andrzej Tarnawski

Chapter 11

Gastroprotection by Nonprostaglandin Substances 197

Stanislaw J. Konturek and Jan W. Konturek

I

Cytoprotection for the Clinician

Cytoprotection
Historical Perspective

ANDRÉ ROBERT

1. INTRODUCTION

Traditionally, the aim of antiulcer therapy has been either to inhibit secretion of gastric acid by parietal cells or neutralize acid that has already been secreted. To this effect, the use of antacids has been, and continues to be, an effective form of treatment, especially for duodenal ulcer. Anticholinergic agents, by inhibiting the action of acetylcholine (ACh), had been used until the mid-1970s, although the occurrence of side effects always prevented administration of adequate doses. The advent of histamine H_2-antagonists, first metiamide, and later cimetidine, ranitidine, and famotidine, led to the administration of strongly antisecretory doses with only minimal side effects and accelerated the healing of peptic ulcer. More recently, omeprazole, a substituted benzimidazole that inhibits (H^+-K^+)-ATPase within the parietal cell canaliculi, was shown to inhibit acid secretion totally and to induce duodenal ulcer healing in 2 weeks.

These developments have further strengthened the concept that in order to heal peptic ulcer and prevent its recurrence, acid secretion must be inhibited and kept low for months or years. Until recently, ulcer therapy has remained focused on the aggressive factors, i.e., acid and pepsin activity, and little attention was paid to the role of mucosal defensive factors. Research on cytoprotection during

ANDRÉ ROBERT • Drug Metabolism Research, The Upjohn Company, Kalamazoo, Michigan 49001.

the past 10 years suggests that natural defensive processes may play a major role in maintaining gastrointestinal integrity.

2. ANTIULCER EFFECT WITHOUT ACID INHIBITION

In 1975, studies by Robert *et al.* suggested that certain forms of gastric ulcerations in rats could be prevented without interfering with acid secretion. In these studies, certain prostaglandins administered either orally or subcutaneously at doses that did not affect acid secretion prevented formation of gastric ulcers produced by a variety of nonsteroidal anti-inflammatory drugs (NSAID). This was the case for some of the natural prostaglandins, such as PGE_2, as well as synthetic prostaglandins, such as $PGEF_{2\beta}$, 15-methyl-PGE_2, and 16,16-dimethyl-PGE_2 (Fig. 1). This finding suggested that certain natural substances, known to be present in the gastric mucosa and gastric juice, could prevent formation of gastric ulcers without interfering with gastric secretion. It was also surmised that the pathogenesis of NSAID-induced ulcers, such as produced by aspirin or indomethacin, may be due to a gastric mucosal depletion of prostaglandins, since NSAID inhibit prostaglandin synthesis. Prevention of NSAID-induced ulcers by exogenous prostaglandins was viewed as the result of replacement therapy in stomachs whose ability to form prostaglandins had been blocked.

The model of NSAID-induced gastric ulcers in animals was not ideal. Although these ulcers were prevented by nonantisecretory doses of prostaglandins, they could also be inhibited by antisecretory agents unrelated to prostaglandins, such as anticholinergic drugs, as well as by antacids. The reason was that NSAID-induced ulcers require some acid within the gastric lumen. Therefore, the choice of this model for studying natural defensive mechanisms as opposed to aggressive factors was not the most appropriate. A search was then started to develop an animal model of gastric mucosal injury that would not respond to inhibitors of acid secretion.

A variety of strong irritants were administered orally to rats in the hope that they would induce necrosis of the gastric mucosa, whether acid was present or not. Severe mucosal lesions were thus produced by oral administration of necrotizing agents. Such agents included absolute ethanol, 0.6 M HCl, 0.2 M NaOH, a hypertonic solution (25% NaCl), and boiling water. The lesions consisted of extensive necrotic areas occupying about one fourth of the gastric mucosa, and penetrating down to four fifths of the mucosa, although not reaching the muscularis mucosae.

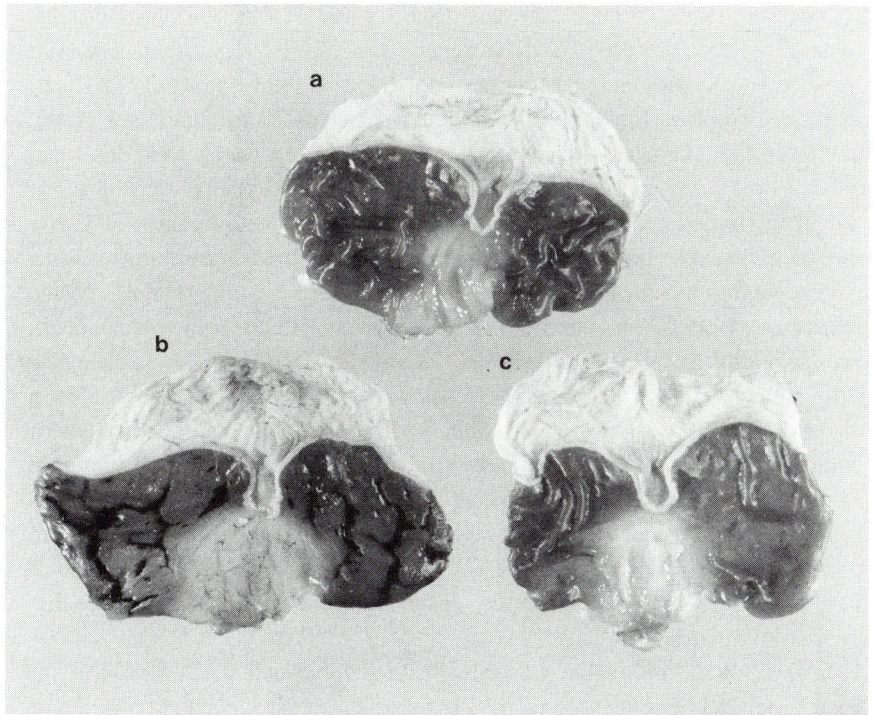

Figure 1. Cytoprotection by a prostaglandin against aspirin-induced gastric ulcers in rats. (a) Normal rat stomach. (b) Severe gastric ulcers produced in 1 h by oral administration of 150 mg/kg aspirin suspended in 0.1 M HCl. (c) Protection of the gastric mucosa by oral treatment with 2.5 μg/kg 15(R)-15-methyl PGE$_2$ (Arbaprostil), a nonantisecretory dose, given 30 min before administration of acidified aspirin.

3. DIRECT CYTOPROTECTION

Using this animal model, the first studies were aimed at determining whether antisecretory agents would prevent the development of mucosal necrosis. None of the antisecretory agents used, i.e., methscopolamine, an anticholinergic agent; cimetidine, a histamine H_2-antagonist; omeprazole, a $[H^+-K^+]$-ATPase inhibitor, prevented the lesions. It was concluded that the mucosal necrosis induced by these agents was not acid dependent. The next question was to determine whether prostaglandins would be protective. At first, antisecretory prostaglandins were administered at doses that inhibited gastric acid secretion; total protection against the necrotizing agents was observed. When lower doses were administered, it was found that extremely low doses of the prostaglandins were still protective. For instance, 16,16-dimethyl-PGE$_2$ inhibited gastric secretion in rats at a dose of 100 μg/kg, whereas it protected the gastric mucosa against absolute ethanol at a dose of 0.5 μg/kg. Obviously, the antisecretory effect was unrelated to the protective effect. Moreover, certain prostaglandins that are not antisecretory at any dose, such as PGF$_{2\beta}$, were also fully protective. When these data were shown to Dr. Eugene D. Jacobson, then at the University of Texas at Houston, he suggested that the phenomenon be called cytoprotection, since the gastric mucosal cells appeared to be protected from necrosis when exposed to prostaglandins. Cytoprotection is defined as the property of substances such as prostaglandins given at nonantisecretory doses to protect the gastric mucosa from becoming necrotic, when this mucosa is exposed to noxious agents. Cytoprotection is separate from, and unrelated to, inhibition of gastric secretion.

At first, the protection was thought to involve the full thickness of the gastric mucosa. Further studies by Lacy and Ito demonstrated two additional facts: (1) in areas of the mucosa that appeared normal with the naked eye, some histological damage to the surface epithelial monolayer covering the mucosa were detected; (2) the gastric mucosa could reconstitute the damaged surface epithelium within a few minutes after exposure to a necrotizing agent by migration of neighboring intact cells. Therefore, the definition of cytoprotection must state that the prevention of necrosis by prostaglandins is directed at cells located under the surface epithelium, and thus involves more than 95% of the mucosal thickness.

Cytoprotection was also demonstrated *in vitro,* using either isolated canine mucosa damaged by indomethacin or frog gastric mucosa damaged by removal of bicarbonate in the incubation medium.

4. DIFFERENCES AMONG PROSTAGLANDINS

Cytoprotection by prostaglandins is obtained at doses that are a fraction of their antisecretory dose, or by prostaglandins that are not antisecretory at any dose. Small doses of prostaglandins also protect the gastric mucosa against the severe lesions produced by aspirin, even when the latter is suspended in increasing concentrations of HCl, whereas antisecretory agents, such as methscopolamine, cimetidine, and omeprazole, are ineffective. Cytoprotective prostaglandins are active after either oral or parenteral administration. The activity is usually three times more marked after the oral route, probably because by this route the full dose is in direct contact with the target organ (the gastric mucosa), whereas after parenteral administration only a portion of the injected dose reaches the stomach via the blood and also undergoes metabolic degradation. The duration of action of cytoprotection depends on the metabolic stability of the prostaglandin. For instance, $16,16$-dimethyl-PGE_2, which has a much longer half-life than PGE_2, is 100 times more cytoprotective; its duration of action is also three to five times longer.

5. CLINICAL STUDIES ON CYTOPROTECTION

Several prostaglandins of the E type were administered orally to human subjects with induced gastric erosions. Thus, PGE_2 prevented occult bleeding from the stomach and endoscopic visual damage caused by aspirin. Oral administration of 40% ethanol produced cellular exfoliation, as measured by the DNA content of gastric washings; oral treatment with PGE_2 prevented such damage. In this study, the cells were held together instead of being shed, and maintained their integrity.

6. ADAPTIVE CYTOPROTECTION

Since several prostaglandins (PGE_2, PGD_2, $PGF_{2\alpha}$, PGI_2) have been identified in the gastric mucosa and gastric juice, it was hypothesized that their formation might contribute to the mucosal integrity seen in healthy subjects, in spite of the presence of the hostile environment of the stomach, characterized by a low pH, the presence of a proteolytic enzyme (pepsin), and the ingestion of indiscriminate foods and liquids at various temperatures and pH values. It was reasoned that the constant presence of prostaglandins in the stomach may exert a cytoprotective effect against these potentially noxious agents.

The possibility that the formation of prostaglandins by the gastric mucosa might be increased by irritating luminal contents was explored. The hypothesis was that certain substances present in the gastric lumen, either naturally or following ingestion, might trigger the synthesis of prostaglandins by the mucosa, and thereby protect the latter from damage if exposed to noxious agents. The role of mild irritants was examined. It was found that a variety of mild irritants (20% ethanol, 0.075 M NaOH, 0.35 M HCl, 4% NaCl, water at 70°C), administered orally to rats, protected the gastric mucosa from necrosis when the stomach was later exposed to very strong irritants, such as absolute ethanol. Since this protection was prevented by prior treatment with indomethacin, an inhibitor of prostaglandin synthesis, it was concluded that mild irritants protected the stomach by stimulating the formation and release of prostaglandins by the stomach. Actual measurement of the generation of prostaglandins by the gastric mucosa supported that hypothesis: several mild irritants did indeed stimulate the formation of prostaglandins by the gastric mucosa. This phenomenon was called adaptive cytoprotection.

Adaptive cytoprotection can occur either when the mild irritant and the necrotizing agent are the same substance (such as protection by 20% ethanol against absolute ethanol), or when the two substances are different (protection by 0.075 M NaOH against necrosis produced by a hypertonic solution such as 25% NaCl). The first phenomenon was called "homocytoprotection," and the second "cross-cytoprotection." Similar studies were performed in dogs in which a low concentration of ethanol (8%) protected the gastric mucosa against a stronger concentration (40% ethanol). Cytoprotection by mild irritants lasts approximately 1 hr. However, repeated administration of a mild irritant such as 0.075 NaOH every hour for 8 hr maintained adaptive cytoprotection for as long as it was given, as shown by challenge with absolute ethanol. In other words, there appears to be no exhaustion in the formation of prostaglandins in response to mild irritants by the stomach.

7. FUNCTIONAL CYTOPROTECTION

The studies reported above demonstrated that prostaglandins, either exogenous (direct cytoprotection) or endogenous (adaptive cytoprotection), can protect the gastric mucosa from necrosis and ulcerations by a mechanism independent of inhibition of acid secretion. In animals given only absolute ethanol, large areas of the parietal cell mass were destroyed; consequently, acid secretion was abolished. Pretreatment with a nonantisecretory dose of prostaglandin not only preserved the integrity of the parietal cells, as seen histologically (morphological cytoprotection), but also maintained the ability of these cells to secrete acid (functional cytoprotection). This was demonstrated by the following experiments.

Rats were given 1 ml absolute ethanol; the pylorus was ligated at various time intervals (from 4 hr to 10 days) after ethanol. The rats were killed 2 hr after pylorus ligation, and the acid content of their gastric juice was measured. Absolute ethanol totally inhibited gastric acid secretion for 8 hr, after which secretion slowly returned to control levels; secretion had recovered to normal baseline only after 2 days. In animals pretreated with 16,16-dimethyl PGE_2, there was only a slight decrease of secretion at 4 hr; thereafter, secretion was normal. Those findings showed that not only do prostaglandins maintain the morphological integrity of gastric parietal cells in spite of the presence of a necrotizing agent, but they also maintain the function of these cells.

8. INTESTINAL CYTOPROTECTION

It has been known for many years that administration of a high dose of NSAID, such as indomethacin, produces within 2–3 days a fatal syndrome of peritonitis in several animal species. Multiple ulcers develop in the jejunum and the ileum; consequently the intestinal mucosa becomes necrotic and the ulcers perforate. At necropsy, abundant peritoneal exudate is present, the intestinal loops are adhesive and often form a solid mass. When it became known that NSAID inhibit prostaglandin cyclo-oxygenase, and therefore block prostaglandin synthesis in tissues, it was hypothesized that this intestinal syndrome might be attributable not to the NSAID themselves, but rather to the prostaglandin deficiency they produce in the intestine. To test this possibility, indomethacin was administered to rats at a dose known to induce intestinal lesions (10 mg/kg). Other animals received the same dose of indomethacin plus prostaglandins in order to compensate for the induced deficiency. The hypothesis proved correct: none of the animals treated with an adequate dose of prostaglandin developed intestinal lesions, in spite of indomethacin treatment. It was concluded that indeed an intestinal prostaglandin deficiency can lead to a severe intestinal syndrome characterized by multiple ulcerations and perforations.

Glucocorticoids, such as prednisolone, inhibit phospholipase A_2 and thereby prevent the release of arachidonic acid from phospholipid pools. Since arachidonic acid is the precursor of prostaglandins, inhibition of phospholipase A_2 by prednisolone can produce a prostaglandin deficiency. Prednisolone was administered to rats daily for 8 days. This led to the formation of intestinal lesions, mostly located in the terminal ileum. Treatment with a prostaglandin such as 16,16-dimethyl PGE_2 prevented such lesions. It was concluded that, as in the case of indomethacin, the intestinal lesions produced by prednisolone were probably mediated through a prostaglandin deficiency, through the inhibition of phospholipase A_2.

Prostaglandins were also studied against other forms of intestinal lesions. Certain antibiotics can stimulate the proliferation of a particular intestinal anaerobic microorganism, *Clostridium difficile*. This microorganism is responsible for antibiotic-associated pseudomembranous colitis that has been observed occasionally in humans. The colitis is caused by the elaboration of a toxin by the microorganism. This disease has been reproduced in hamsters by administration of certain broad-spectrum antibiotics. In this species, colitis is limited to the cecum (cecitis). When certain prostaglandins were given to antibiotic-treated animals, the cecitis was prevented. It was concluded that intestinal cytoprotection extends to the large intestine. Another model of intestinal lesion consists of introducing ethanol into the colon of rats. This leads to acute colitis. Pretreatment with 16,16-dimethyl PGE_2 markedly reduced the severity of the colitis.

9. CONCLUSIONS

Prostaglandins are cytoprotective for the stomach and for the small and the large intestine. The mechanism of cytoprotection is unknown but is unrelated to an effect on gastric acid secretion. The demonstration that the gastric mucosa can be protected from necrosis by agents that do not reduce acid secretion suggests that acid does not always play a role in the development of gastric injury. A distinction can be made between antiulcer agents (acting primarily through the inhibition of acid secretion) and cytoprotective agents (acting in spite of the presence of gastric acid) (Fig. 2).

The protective effect of prostaglandins, which are natural substances, suggests that these compounds may contribute to the natural defense of the gastric mucosa against ulcerogenic agents. The use of such protective agents can be anticipated, either prostaglandins or other compounds that have also been shown to be protective, to be used in the treatment of gastrointestinal diseases in which mucosal injury is the primary defect.

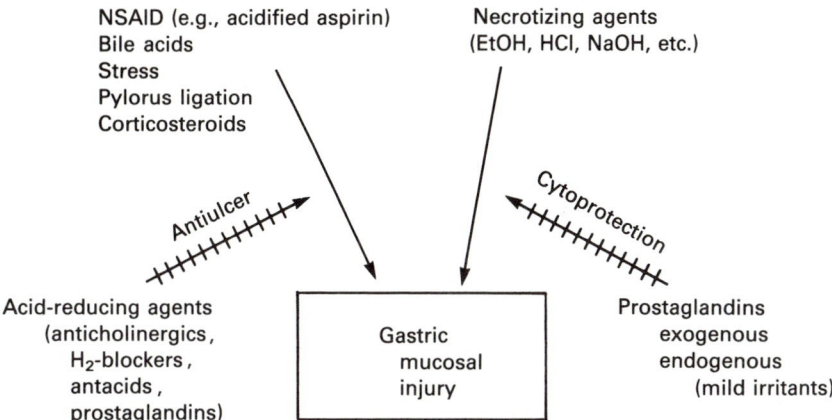

Figure 2. Distinction between antiulcer and cytoprotective activities. NSAID, nonsteroidal anti-inflammatory drugs. (From Robert *et al.*, 1984.)

ANNOTATED BIBLIOGRAPHY

Guth PH, Paulsen G, Nagata H: Histologic and microcirculatory changes in alcohol-induced gastric lesions in the rat: Effect of prostaglandin cytoprotection. *Gastroenterology* **87:**1083–1090, 1984.

These studies show that cytoprotective prostaglandins maintain the microcirculation of the gastric mucosa, even after exposure to ethanol.

Lacy ER, Ito S: Microscopic analysis of ethanol damage to rat gastric mucosa after treatment with a prostaglandin, *Gastroenterology* **83:**619–625, 1982.

Prostaglandin protects the gastric mucosa from necrosis after exposure to ethanol, while the surface epithelium is not protected; rapid mucosal restitution by cell migration is described.

Robert A: Antisecretory, antiulcer, cytoprotective, and diarrheogenic properties of prostaglandins. *Adv Prostaglandins Thromboxane Res* 507–520, 1976.

This is the first report on the gastric and intestinal cytoprotective effect of prostaglandins.

Robert A: Cytoprotection by prostaglandins. *Gastroenterology* **77:**761–67, 1979.

This paper reviews the various types of cytoprotection, gastric and intestinal.

Robert A, Nezamis JE, Lancaster C, et al: Mild irritants prevent gastric necrosis through "adaptive cytoprotection" mediated by prostaglandins. *Am J Physiol* **245:**G113–121, 1983.

These studies show that adaptive cytoprotection can be produced by mild irritants, via stimulation of endogenous formation of prostaglandins by the stomach.

Schmidt KL, Henagan JM, Hilburn PJ, et al: Prostaglandin cytoprotection against ethanol-induced gastric injury in the rat: A histologic and cytologic study of the surface epithelium. *Gastroenterology* **88:**649–659, 1985.

This light and electron microscopic study describes gastric mucosal lesions produced by ethanol, as well as the extent of protection by a prostaglandin.

Szabo S, Trier JS, Frankel PW: Sulfhydryl compounds may mediate gastric cytoprotection. *Science* **214**:200–202, 1981.

This article presents studies on the role of sulfhydryl compounds in the mechanism of gastric cytoprotection.

Tarnawski A, Hollander D, Stachura J, et al: Prostaglandin protection of the gastric mucosa against alcohol injury—A dynamic time-related process. Role of the mucosal proliferative zone. *Gastroenterology* **88**:344–352, 1985.

This article describes a light and electron microscopic study of gastric mucosal cytoprotection by a prostaglandin in function of time, showing that the mucosal proliferative zone is protected.

Terano A, Mach T, Stachura J, et al: Effect of 16,16-dimethyl prostaglandin E_2 on aspirin-induced damage to gastric epithelial cells in tissue culture. *Gut* **25**:19–25, 1984.

This study shows that a prostaglandin applied *in vitro* to cultured gastric cells reduces damage produced by aspirin.

Whittle BJR, Steel G: Evaluation of the protection of rat gastric mucosa by a prostaglandin analogue using cellular enzyme marker and histologic techniques. *Gastroenterology* **88**:315–327, 1984.

A cytoprotective prostaglandin protects gastric mucosal cells against ethanol, as shown by the prevention of release of cellular enzymes and by histology.

2

Acid Hypersecretion
Important Factor or Innocent Bystander?

JAMES PENSTON and KENNETH G. WORMSLEY

1. INTRODUCTION

Peptic ulcers are discrete wounds of the mucosa of the esophagus, stomach, and duodenum or, following gastric surgery, of the small intestine which has been anastomosed to the stomach. Peptic ulcers have the common attribute of occurring only in those parts of the alimentary tract which are exposed to gastric secretions. This feature, together with the demonstration that gastric juice has the capacity to destroy animal tissues, has resulted in the belief that peptic ulceration is, in some way, caused by exposure of the affected mucosa to gastric secretions.

Duodenal ulcers are, in most countries and during the twentieth century, the most common type of ulcer to affect the upper alimentary tract and consequently have been studied in most detail. This chapter presents an analysis of the evidence linking gastric secretion, and especially gastric hypersecretion, with the pathogenesis of duodenal ulcers.

JAMES PENSTON and KENNETH G. WORMSLEY • Ninewells Hospital, Dundee DD1 9SY, Scotland.

2. INFORMATION INTERPRETED AS INDICATING A CONNECTION BETWEEN GASTRIC JUICE AND DUODENAL ULCERATION

2.1. Animal Studies

Surgical manipulation of the upper alimentary tract of animals has been used to create models for the investigation of duodenal ulcer disease. Operations that divert the flow of gastric juice directly into the jejunum or ileum (Mann–Williamson procedure) result in ulceration of the small intestine that has been anastomosed to the stomach. Under an apparently different set of conditions, gastric and duodenal ulcers develop when the gastric antrum is transplanted to the transverse colon. Unfortunately, interpretation of these studies in terms of the noxious effects of gastric juice is difficult, since the operations involve gross distortion of the anatomy and physiology of the upper alimentary tract.

Subsequent studies have therefore avoided operative intervention and have, instead, involved the introduction into the animal's stomach or small intestine of some, or all, of the components of gastric juice, thus simulating sustained gastric hypersecretion. Alternatively, the animals have been stimulated to secrete gastric juice in abnormally large amounts and for prolonged periods of time by the parenteral administration of gastric secretagogues or by the administration of ulcerogens such as cysteamine. In an example of one such study, intragastric administration of 0.1 M HCl plus pepsin to dogs produced duodenal ulcers, but only if the animals also developed metabolic acidosis. Parenteral administration of sodium bicarbonate prevented the development of duodenal ulcers even if the substitute gastric juice was instilled continuously for 5 days. If the strength of the acid was increased to 0.15 M, however, intravenous bicarbonate did not prevent the development of gastric or duodenal ulcers.

Parenteral administration of gastric secretagogues has elicited duodenal ulcers in a number of different species. Injection of histamine, especially in slow-release preparations, produces duodenal ulcers in rats, guinea pigs, cats, and dogs. Subcutaneous and intravenous gastrin and pentagastrin also produce duodenal ulcers in rats, guinea pigs, and cats, while the combination of subcutaneous pentagastrin and carbachol results in a 100% incidence of duodenal ulcers in rats.

The results of these different types of animal studies are compatible with the view that excessive amounts of gastric juice have an etiologic role in the pathogenesis of duodenal ulcers and confirm that intraluminal infusion of solutions containing both acid and pepsin are more ulcerogenic than solutions containing only acid.

2.2. Human Studies

Data held to provide evidence that excessive or inappropriate amounts of gastric juice are involved in ulcerogenesis include the following studies.

2.2.1. Experiments of Nature

In humans, several disease states can be viewed as experiments of nature that apparently shed light on the relationship between gastric secretion and the development of duodenal ulceration. The best example of an association between secretion of abnormally large amounts of gastric juice and a high incidence of duodenal ulcers is provided by the Zollinger–Ellison syndrome, which is characterized by severe duodenal ulceration in more than 90% of affected patients. The ulcers can be healed and maintained in remission by therapeutic suppression of gastric secretion or by resection of the stomach. Patients with chronic renal failure, treated with dialysis, suffer almost as high (more than 50%) an incidence of duodenal ulcers.

A very high incidence of jejunal ulcers is also observed after gastrojejunostomy, especially when the gastric antrum has been separated from the stomach and left in continuity with the duodenum (retained antrum syndrome). Meckel's diverticulum is sometimes accompanied by ulceration of the ileum opposite the diverticulum. The diverticulum in these patients contains ectopic gastric mucosa, which has been shown to secrete acid.

Conversely, to be set against these examples of ulcers associated with increased or inappropriate secretion of gastric juice, it seems that duodenal ulcers never occur in patients with achlorhydria which has usually resulted from atrophic gastritis or gastric atrophy, as a result of the disappearance of the gastric parietal and chief cells and consequent loss of the capacity to secrete gastric juice. The strength of the association between absence of gastric juice and absence of duodenal ulceration has given rise to Schwarz's dictum: "No acid, no ulcer."

2.2.2. Gastric Secretion in Patients with Idiopathic Duodenal Ulcers

In patients with duodenal ulcer, the secretion of gastric juice has been studied in the unstimulated stomach (in the form of basal, interdigestive, and nocturnal secretion) and in response to gastric secretagogues. Basal and nocturnal gastric secretion is increased in many patients with duodenal ulcer. The latter form of inappropriate secretion is considered especially important in the development of duodenal ulcers. In addition, the gastric response to all secretory stimulants is higher in a proportion of duodenal ulcer patients (15–40%, depending on secretory stimulus) than in any control subjects, giving rise to higher average levels of gastric secretion when groups of patients with duodenal ulcer are compared with nonulcer controls. In response to the stimulus of food, however, the average gastric secretory response of duodenal ulcer patients is generally not increased, although the duration of the secretory response is often prolonged compared with control subjects. Thus, the 24-hr gastric secretion of acid has been reported to be twice as great in a group of patients with duodenal ulcer as in control subjects.

In summary, patients with duodenal ulcer have higher average values of unstimulated and secretagogue-induced gastric secretion than do control subjects, but most ulcer patients do not suffer from any form of gastric hypersecretion. Nevertheless, admittedly, very few patients with duodenal ulcer have had all aspects of gastric secretion studied or compared with nonulcer patients.

2.2.3. Factors Predisposing to Increased Gastric Secretion

Many pathophysiologic abnormalities have been described and thought to account for the increased gastric secretion of patients with duodenal ulcer. The number of parietal cells (size of parietal cell mass) has been reported to be increased in patients with duodenal ulcer. Increased parietal cell mass has been considered to explain the increased gastric secretory response to stimulants in patients with duodenal ulcer.

By contrast, the tendency to secrete excessive amounts of gastric juice inappropriately (i.e., between meals and at night, when there is apparently no specific stimulus to secretion) has been explained by the finding that the sensitivity of the parietal cells to endogenous and exogenous stimulants is increased in some patients with duodenal ulcer. One such endogenous gastric secretory stimulus is provided by the increased levels of circulating gastrin described in patients with duodenal ulcer, both in the basal state and after food consumption. Similarly, an increased secretory response to gastric distention has been recorded in ulcer patients. These latter phenomena might be expected to account for relatively greater than normal rates of gastric secretion at submaximal levels of stimulation and could account for the more prolonged gastric secretory response to food in patients with duodenal ulcer.

In addition to the increased capacity for, and stimulation of, gastric secretion in patients with duodenal ulcer, it has also been reported that the inhibitory influence on the stomach of these patients is defective. For example, it has been suggested that the feedback inhibition of gastric secretion by acid in the antrum or duodenum is less in ulcer patients than in control subjects, a circumstance which may also result in 'inappropriate' gastric secretion.

2.2.4. Duodenal Acidity

If excess gastric juice is involved in the development of duodenal ulcers, the amount of acid or the duration of exposure of the duodenal bulb to acid must be greater in ulcer patients than in controls. Studies to assess duodenal bulbar pH have given contradictory results. Some studies have shown increased duodenal acidity in ulcer patients, compared with control subjects, while others have shown much, or complete, overlap between the values of bulbar pH of the two groups, indicating that many patients with duodenal ulcer have duodenal bulbar acidity similar to that of nonulcer patients.

2.2.5. Factors Predisposing to Abnormally Acid Duodenal Bulbar pH

Increased rates of discharge of gastric contents into the duodenum (increased rates of gastric emptying) might be expected to increase the acid load delivered into the duodenal bulb. Such increased rates of gastric emptying have been recorded in patients with duodenal ulcer, as has increased delivery of acid into the duodenum.

Excessive amounts of acid in the duodenal bulb may also result from defective removal of acid from the duodenal lumen. In this connection, it has been reported that patients with duodenal ulcer secrete less than normal amounts of bicarbonate into the duodenum, resulting in decreased buffering of the intraluminal acid. The decreased bicarbonate secretion has been attributed both to decreased release of secretin from the small intestinal mucosa and to decreased production of prostaglandins in the duodenal mucosa following exposure to acid. It has also been reported that the motility of the proximal duodenum is defective in patients with duodenal ulcer, so that potentially noxious contents are not cleared satisfactorily.

2.3. Response to Treatment

Evidence that gastric juice is involved in the etiology of ulcers is also provided by the response to therapeutic removal of acid and by therapeutic inhibition of gastric secretion. Drugs exhibiting these effects have been shown to heal ulcers and, when treatment is continued after ulcer healing, to maintain remission of the ulcers. Indeed, the therapeutic inhibition of gastric secretion has been so successful in healing ulcers, that this aspect of alimentary function is used as the principal criterion for assessing the potential efficacy of new antiulcer drugs.

2.3.1. Antiulcer Drugs

Antacids have been shown to increase significantly the rate of healing of duodenal ulcers. Antacids have long been assumed to exert their therapeutic effects by buffering acid and thereby inactivating pepsin, although recently the doses of antacids used to heal ulcers have become so small that the buffering capacity of the ingested antacid is no longer adequate to dispose of more than a small fraction of the acid secreted by most patients with duodenal ulcer. The mechanism whereby antacids heal ulcers remain to be defined.

The currently used histamine H_2-receptor antagonists heal 60–80% of duodenal ulcers after treatment for 4 weeks, while the rate of healing is more than 90% after treatment for 8 weeks. Continuous treatment, with night-time administration of the drugs, has kept duodenal ulcers in remission for more than 10 years. Full doses of H_2-receptor antagonists inhibit gastric secretion by about 70%, while night-time therapy inhibits nocturnal secretion to a similar, or greater, extent but does not affect daytime secretion of gastric juice.

Omeprazole, a proton pump blocker, is an even more powerful inhibitor of gastric secretion. The output of gastric juice can be virtually abolished by treatment with the drug for a week or so. Omeprazole, in a dose that abolishes gastric secretion, heals all or nearly all duodenal ulcers within 4 weeks of treatment. Anticholinergic drugs, such as pirenzepine and telenzepine, are weaker inhibitors of gastric secretion but heal about 70% of duodenal ulcers during 4 weeks of treatment.

2.3.2. Gastric Surgery

In addition to the therapeutic efficacy of gastric inhibitory drugs, gastric operations have long been used in an attempt to heal duodenal ulcers and to keep ulcers in remission. For example, after vagotomy and antrectomy, virtually abolishing the gastric secretory response to stimulants, the rate of recurrence of ulcers is as low as 1%. By contrast, highly selective vagotomy is followed by recurrence rates of 30% or more, the recurrences occurring especially in patients whose gastric response to stimulants has decreased by less than 60% compared with preoperative values.

In summary, it seems that therapeutic measures that inhibit gastric secretion increase the healing of duodenal ulcers and maintain remission. It also appears that the success of therapy in healing ulcers is related to the ability of the drug or operation to inhibit gastric secretion. It is not clear, though, why the very limited inhibition of gastric secretion provided by nocturnal treatment regimens is so effective in healing ulcers and keeping ulcers in remission.

2.4. Relationship between Acid and Pepsin in Gastric Juice

There is a close relationship between the secretion of acid and pepsin, since most stimulants of acid secretion also stimulate the secretion of pepsinogen. Thus, as with the output of acid, patients with duodenal ulcer secrete, on average, increased amounts of pepsin compared with controls. When gastric secretion is markedly inhibited so, generally, is the secretion of pepsin. In our discussion of the role of gastric juice in the pathogenesis of ulcers, it is therefore assumed that reference to acid means acid plus pepsin, in view of the parallelism of secretion of these two components of gastric juice under most circumstances.

3. ANALYSIS OF THE EVIDENCE FOR THE ROLE OF GASTRIC SECRETION IN ULCEROGENESIS

3.1. Animal Studies

The Mann–Williamson and other types of operation used to produce experimental ulcers almost invariably produce sustained gastric hypersecretion as a result of severe disturbances of function of the upper alimentary tract. While the gastric hypersecretion is easy to identify and explain (being the result of sustained inappropriate stimulation of secretion, defective inhibition of secretion, and hyperplasia of the parietal cells) and, while excessive exposure to gastric juice may be involved in the etiology of the associated ulcers, it is interesting (and probably very significant, from the point of view of the etiology of ulcers) that intestinal and other tissues transplanted directly into the stomach do not ulcerate. These findings were interpreted as showing that pure gastric juice had corrosive properties, while normal gastric contents were more or less innocuous, unless present in very large amounts. The latter hypothesis cannot be tested or proved but seems inherently improbable. Surprisingly, no attention has been paid to the other, nongastric functional abnormalities that also result from the experimental surgery and that may be more relevant than gastric juice to the etiology of postoperative ulcers.

In an early comprehensive analysis of the etiologic implications of gastric juice in ulcerogenesis, it was proposed that the role of gastric juice could best be assessed by analyzing the consequences of the experimental removal of physiologic antagonists of gastric secretion and by studying the effects of production of excessive amounts of gastric juice. The former studies involved the production of ulcer by interference with the normal drainage of protective bile and pancreatic juice into the duodenum or excluding the duodenum with its protective secretions from normal alimentary continuity. In dogs, all these procedures resulted in the production of ulcers. However, the health of the animals invariably deteriorated as a result of severe disturbances of alimentary function and digestion. In view of the difficulties encountered in attempting to interpret the complex postoperative conditions of the animals, secretagogues were used to produce gastric hypersecretion and resulted in a high incidence of ulcers of the duodenum. It was concluded that the most important single factor in ulcerogenesis was the hypersecretion of acid gastric juice. It has been repeatedly shown, however, that (histamine-induced) gastric hypersecretion only delays, but does not prevent, the healing of (traumatic) ulcers. In any case, it should not be assumed that secretagogues are ulcerogenic only as a result of stimulating gastric hypersecretion. Thus, histamine has been reported to exert angiotoxic effects and also to inhibit repair of wounds directly, even under *in vitro* conditions (i.e., even in the absence of gastric juice).

In summary, the animal studies are most easily interpreted as indicating that abnormally large amounts of gastric juice are etiologically involved in the development of duodenal (and small intestinal) ulcers. However, all recorded types of study are fundamentally complex, and their interpretation in terms of the etiologic involvement of acid in ulcerogenesis is therefore potentially (and actually) flawed. Moreover, even when animal studies have shown that instillation of acid and pepsin produces duodenal ulcers, the quantities of the simulated gastric juice required to produce the ulcers are greatly in excess of normally secreted amounts of gastric juice. These studies therefore cannot, and do not, define the role of normal amounts of gastric juice in the production of ulcers.

3.2. Human Studies

3.2.1. Experiments of Nature

The association of gastric hypersecretion and duodenal ulceration that characterizes Zollinger–Ellison syndrome has been interpreted as supporting the implications of the animal studies. That is, it has been assumed that the continuous exposure of the duodenal mucosa to large amounts of gastric juice causes the duodenal and small intestinal ulceration. It is important to note, however, that gastric ulceration is very uncommon in patients with Zollinger–Ellison syndrome (and, indeed, some patients with the syndrome suffer from no intestinal ulceration at all, despite the gastric hypersecretion). The apparent resistance of the gastric (and sometimes duodenal) mucosa to the very large amounts of gastric juice has not been explained. Another point of interest is the finding that the duodenal ulcers associated with Zollinger–Ellison syndrome heal following the administration of gastric secretory inhibitors, although the degree of residual gastric hypersecretion (as much as 10 mmoles/hr basal secretion) remains much greater than the basal secretion of most patients with active idiopathic duodenal ulcers. It should therefore be emphasized that the alterations in alimentary function and the maldigestion that characterizes Zollinger–Ellison syndrome resemble the disturbances encountered in dogs after ulcer-producing operations. While it is permissible to conclude that severe gastric hypersecretion can produce duodenal ulcers, these observations do not preclude the pathogenic role of other functional disturbances. More important, the findings in Zollinger–Ellison syndrome do not permit inferences about the causal role of gastric secretions in the development of duodenal ulcers in patients whose output of gastric juice is less than that of patients with gastrinomas.

During dialysis, the hypergastrinemia associated with chronic renal failure results in sustained gastric hypersecretion and associated disturbance of alimentary function similar to those of patients with gastrinomas. While the levels of gastric secretion are not as great, the sustained hypergastrinemia of patients with the retained antrum syndrome also produces continuous exposure of the jejunal mucosa to inappropriate amounts of gastric juice. However, as with animal studies, the underlying disturbance of the normal anatomy and function of the upper alimentary tract make it difficult to interpret the etiologic basis of the associated ulceration.

The etiology of the ulceration associated with Meckel's diverticulum is also unclear, not only because the characteristics and magnitude of the acid secretion have not been defined, but also because the ectopic gastric mucosa may represent a metaplastic reaction to small intestinal ulceration, such as is observed in the duodenal mucosa around duodenal ulcers.

3.2.2. Gastric Secretion in Patients with Duodenal Ulcer

While the average values of gastric secretion (or other aspects of alimentary function are greater than normal in patients with duodenal ulcer, apparently most of these patients are functionally not different from control subjects; thus, only a small proportion of ulcer patients show an increase in one of the measured indices of function which are considered to be etiologically involved in ulcerogenesis.

In assessing the hypothesis that gastric hypersecretion causes duodenal ulcers, it must be emphasized that the categorisation of control groups as normal may be misleading, since the subjects in the control groups are usually neither examined endoscopically nor followed clinically to ensure that they do not develop ulcers. Since it is not yet possible to identify a predisposition to duodenal ulceration, it is likely that control groups include persons who have had, or who suffer from, or who will develop duodenal ulcers. Conversely, it is not certain that study of gastric secretion at a certain point in time necessarily reflects the gastric function of ulcer patients. For example, it has been reported that, during environmental stress, ulcer-prone persons may develop gastric hypersecretion which, it has been assumed, is etiologically involved in the development of their ulcer. (In this connection, it is not known whether stress similarly provokes gastric hypersecretion in nonulcer persons in whom an ulcer does not subsequently develop.)

Equally important, there is as yet no agreement about which index of gastric function must be used to define patients with duodenal ulcer. It is possible that different patterns of gastric hypersecretion are etiologically important in different patients, but there remain no practical or theoretical bases for resolving the problem.

While all the available evidence is compatible with the hypothesis that gastric hypersecretion is the cause of some duodenal ulcers, it seems that most ulcer patients do not secrete excessive amounts of gastric juice. In these patients, if secretory studies do reflect the gastric secretory status, gastric hypersecretion cannot be the cause of the duodenal ulcers, although some role for (normal amounts of) gastric juice in the pathogenesis of the duodenal ulcers cannot be excluded. Under these circumstances, however, factors other than gastric juice must be involved in the etiology of the ulcers, since apparently identical amounts of gastric juice do not cause ulcers in control (nonulcer) subjects. In normally secreting ulcer patients, gastric juice is therefore either acting as a permissive factor in ulcerogenesis or is not involved in the etiology of ulcers at all.

3.2.3. Factors Predisposing to Increased Gastric Secretion

The functional abnormalities identified in some patients with duodenal ulcer have been interpreted as supporting the pathogenic role of gastric juice. If gastric juice is involved in ulcerogenesis, that interpretation may be valid. However, it is also possible that the changes in gastric function merely represent paraphenomena; i.e., it is possible that the disorder that causes the duodenal ulceration also disturbs other aspects of the function of the upper alimentary tract (the most easily measured of which is the secretion of gastric juice). Alternatively, the gastric secretory abnormalities may actually be secondary to, and a consequence of, the duodenal ulceration.

There is some evidence from animal experiments for the view that ulcerogenic agents can also produce pathophysiologic disturbances. For example, cysteamine produces duodenal ulcers in rats and also produces nearly all the pathophysiologic disturbances identified in humans with ulcer disease. It has been proposed that in cysteamine-treated rats, as in human subjects, the duodenal ulceration is secondary to the pathophysiologic disturbances, but since the pathologic alterations of the duodenal mucosa precede the pathophysiologic changes, it is reasonable to interpret the occurrence of cysteamine-induced ulcers and of the associated alterations in gastric and duodenal function as reflecting the actions of a common causal agent which is producing these two types of sequelae.

3.2.4. Duodenal Acidity

The most detailed recent studies of intraduodenal pH have shown identical ranges of values in patients with duodenal ulcer and in control subjects. It appears that (1) the intraduodenal pH is normal in patients with duodenal ulcer; (2) the control population appears to be made up of many persons suffering from a duodenal ulcer diathesis; (3) some other functional abnormalities, in addition to the normally low pH transients, are responsible for the duodenal damage caused by gastric juice in the duodenal bulb; or (4) gastric juice is not involved in the development of duodenal ulcers.

3.3. Response to Treatment

A range of drugs and a number of gastric surgical procedures that reduce gastric secretion also increase the rate of healing of ulcers and reduce the rate of recurrence, if treatment with the drugs is continued. It has been suggested that the rate of healing of ulcers is proportional to the degree of gastric inhibition, although other studies have failed to demonstrate any relationship between gastric secretory inhibition and ulcer healing. In general, the satisfactory results of ulcer therapy have been interpreted as indicating that gastric juice is involved in ulcerogenesis and that reduction of duodenal exposure to gastric juice is responsible for healing the ulcers. While it is true that very powerful gastric inhibitors such as omeprazole heal ulcers very rapidly, the evidence linking gastric inhibition with ulcer healing is not wholly convincing, because such gastric operations as highly selective vagotomy reduce gastric secretion by only about 60% but heal virtually all ulcers and keep most ulcers in permanent remission. Similarly, current ulcer-healing regimens with H_2-receptor antagonists heal 95% or more of ulcers but do not influence gastric secretion at all during daytime. It has therefore been necessary to consider alternative explanations for the success or failure of antiulcer therapy.

We have previously proposed that the mechanisms by which all types of antiulcer treatment heal duodenal ulcers may be quite independent of changes in intragastric or intraduodenal acidity. For example, cimetidine has been noted to possess antiviral activity and also to stimulate wound repair directly *in vitro* (in the absence of gastric juice), in addition to its antisecretory effects. The mechanism of the antiulcer effect of cimetidine therefore depends on the (as yet undefined) etiology of the ulcers. Indeed, any apparent relationship between therapeutic gastric inhibition and ulcer-healing efficacy may be spurious and may merely indicate that, for example, antiulcer drugs are actively exerting pharmacologic effects.

Moreover, it is clear that reduction of intragastric acidity is not necessary to control ulcer disease, because such drugs as carbenoxolone, sucralfate, and colloidal bismuth subcitrate, which do not significantly lessen the amounts of acid in the gastric lumen, also heal ulcers and maintain ulcer remission.

In summary, from the point of view of the etiology of ulcers, the efficacy of antiulcer therapy can be interpreted either as indicating that gastric juice in normal or increased amounts is necessary for ulcerogenesis, or alternatively that antiulcer drugs and surgery exert effects that have not yet been definitively identified.

3.4. Relationship between Acid and Pepsin

Much of the discussion of ulcerogenesis is devoted to the noxious effects of gastric acid. Indeed, it has been specifically stated that it is the acid, rather than the pepsin of gastric juice, that produces ulcers. However, much of the evidence for the importance of acid in ulcerogenesis merely reflects the ease with which this latter component of gastric juice can be measured.

In animal experiments, duodenal ulcers have been produced by the instillation of solutions containing both acid and pepsin into the duodenum. In contrast, infusion of acid alone does not produce ulcers. Similarly, it has been shown that gastric distention with an acid solution does not produce gastric ulcers in rats, while the addition of pepsin results in ulceration under these circumstances.

These findings emphasize the potential etiologic importance of pepsin in ulcerogenesis. In this connection, it is necessary to remember that pepsin is an acid protease that loses much of its proteolytic potency at pH levels >3. Since HCl and pepsin are usually secreted in parallel, it seems likely that the principal role of acid is to provide an appropriate milieu for the proteolytic activity of pepsin. When the aggressive nature of acid is discussed, it must therefore be understood that gastric juice, containing both HCl and pepsin, is being considered.

3.5. Heterogeneity

It has recently been suggested that the different pathophysiologic disturbances identified in patients with duodenal ulcer indicate that these patients represent an etiologically heterogeneous group of persons and that duodenal ulceration has multifactorial causation. The subdivision of duodenal ulcers into etiologic subgroups may be correct because duodenal ulcers, like cutaneous wounds, may depict a common pathologic endpoint of different disease processes. However, concepts such as heterogeneity and multifactorial often reflect our ignorance, rather than insight, as was the case in the discussions of the etiology of tuberculosis before the isolation of the causative bacterium. These concepts disappear when more specific etiologic factors are identified.

3.6. Mucosal Injury

In addition to involvement in the etiology of chronic ulcers, it has also been proposed that gastric juice, and, specifically, gastric acid, is involved in the acute breakdown of the gastric and duodenal mucosa. In this connection, it has been shown that acid promotes acute ulcerogenesis when the gastric mucosa is exposed to nonsteroidal anti-inflammatory drugs (NSAID) and when animals or human subjects are exposed to stressful conditions.

However, the etiologic role of gastric juice under the latter circumstances is as difficult to define as in the case of chronic ulcers. For example, NSAID produce ulcers not only in the stomach and duodenum, but also in the small and large intestine, where gastric juice is not present usually. Similarly, it has been claimed that luminal acid plays a negligible role in the genesis of stress-induced gastroduodenal disease in rats. Moreover, it seems possible that intragastric neutralization with antacids lessens the occurrence of stress ulcers not by countering the noxious effects of gastric juice, but rather by preventing mucosal damage as a result of some other effect of the drugs (such as the stimulation of prostaglandin synthesis).

4. ASSOCIATION AND CAUSATION

The problems in determining the cause of chronic diseases have recently been the subject of considerable discussion. Using some of the recommended criteria, we attempt an analysis of the hypothesis that gastric juice—in either increased amounts or normal quantities—causes duodenal ulcers.

4.1. Strength of Association

This criterion refers to the degree of association and to the occurrence of a positive dose–response relationship. In experimental animals, gastric hypersecretion produced by gastric surgery or by secretagogues is often followed by duodenal ulceration. In humans, most patients with gastric hypersecretion resulting from Zollinger–Ellison syndrome develop duodenal ulcers. It seems, therefore, that there is a strong association between experimental and clinical conditions that manifest with gastric hypersecretion and the development of duodenal ulcers (although the converse is not true).

In animals, normal gastric secretion does not cause ulcers. Ulcers can be produced in the duodenum by chemicals which do not alter gastric secretion (e.g., NSAID). In humans, most normal secretors do not suffer from duodenal ulcers, although this statement has not been rigorously tested. For example, in a recent study of asymptomatic volunteers, 2% were found to have asymptomatic duodenal ulcers at the time of endoscopy. Most patients (approximately 75%) with duodenal ulcers secrete normal amounts of gastric juice.

Patients who do not secrete acid do not suffer from duodenal ulcers. If gastric secretion is inhibited to approximately 30% of pretreatment values by therapeutic gastric inhibitors, most ulcers heal. Drugs that completely inhibit gastric secretion heal all ulcers. However, 30–70% of ulcers also heal without active therapy (and therefore presumably without significant change in gastric secretory status).

In summary, it seems that, in all known instances of duodenal ulceration, the hypothetical cause (some gastric juice) and the disease coexist. By contrast, the cause (gastric juice) is not specific in producing the disease, since most people secrete gastric juice without suffering from duodenal ulcers.

A dose–response relationship between secretion of gastric juice and the development of duodenal ulcers also exists, as gastric hypersecretion is associated with a high incidence of duodenal ulcers, while duodenal ulcers are not found in hyposecretors. However, these extremes (gastrinomas and pernicious anemia) result from, and reflect, profound disturbances in the homeostasis of the affected individuals, so that the relevance of the abnormalities of the output of gastric juice to the etiology of the associated ulcer disease remains to be established. Similarly, while the acid-lowering effect of therapeutic measures is compatible with the proposed etiologic role of gastric juice, these measures (gastric inhibitory drugs and gastric surgery) also have effects other than the reduction of gastric secretion so that the etiologic implications of antiulcer therapy are not yet fully understood.

4.2. Consistency of Observed Association

Can the relationship be replicated when studied in different locations by different methods? It has often been shown that in different parts of the world, patients with duodenal ulcers secrete different amounts of gastric juice. For example, Oriental patients with duodenal ulcer secrete about one half as much acid as do Occidental patients. However, gastric hypersecretion is uncommon in patients with idiopathic duodenal ulcers, irrespective of geographic area or historical period.

It has also been pointed out that care must be taken to ensure that the association between the hypothetic cause and the disease is not attributable to some constant error or fallacy. The limitations of the measurement and definition of gastric hypersecretion have been discussed above. Clearly, attributing duodenal ulcers to gastric hypersecretion is quantitatively not correct in most patients and can only be justified by assuming qualitative gastric hypersecretion. That is, it is usually assumed that the gastric secretion of patients with duodenal ulcer, whatever its magnitude, is excessive relative to hypothetic protective or defensive factors (which must therefore be defective in normosecreting ulcer patients). The latter assumptions are usually unstated and always unsubstantiated and may be consistently wrong.

From a different point of view, it has been assumed, with apparently more justification, that the secretion of (some) gastric juice is necessary for the development of duodenal ulcers, because these ulcers do not occur in achlorhydric patients. That observed association may, indeed, denote etiologic involvement of gastric juice in ulcerogenesis. The secretion of gastric juice is the only easily measurable criterion of gastric function, however. It is therefore possible that the apparent association between the secretion of gastric juice and the development of ulcers merely reflects a more profound etiologic relationship between some other aspect of alimentary function and ulcerogenesis—an aspect that has not yet been defined (just as mucus was held to protect the gastric mucosa before it became possible to measure prostaglandins).

4.3. Specificity of Association

This criterion depends on the concept of the distinctiveness of the relationship between the proposed cause and the disease. The suspected etiologic agent is specifically related to the disease, if a similar relationship does not exist with other suspected etiologic factors. The less the frequency of other associations, the higher the specificity of the observed association and the higher the validity of the causal inference (i.e., that gastric juice, and especially the hypersecretion of gastric juice, is involved in causing ulcer disease).

In this connection, until recently no other potential causal associations had been seriously considered. However, other possible etiologic agents, such as viral or bacterial infections, chemical ulcerogens, and pancreatic proteases, are now being studied, but their ulcerogenic potential and relevance have not yet been satisfactorily assessed.

4.4. Temporality

It has been concluded that, in order to confirm a causal relationship, exposure to the alleged cause must precede the development of the alleged effect. While we accept that the ability to secrete some gastric juice always precedes the onset of ulcer disease, it has never been shown that gastric hypersecretion precedes the onset of duodenal ulceration. Satisfactory prospective studies are not available, but clinical follow-up studies of patients some years after gastric secretory studies indicate that those in whom duodenal ulcers develop tend to secrete within the upper range of normal. By contrast, it has also been proposed that gastric hypersecretion is the result of the duodenal ulceration, as serial examination of gastric secretory capacity has demonstrated an increase with the duration of the ulcer disease.

4.5. Plausibility and Coherence

It has been concluded that the relationship between the proposed cause and disease must not conflict with known facts about the biology of the disease.

Unfortunately, too little is known about the normal functions of the upper alimentary tract and its disorders in ulcer disease to permit assessment of this criterion in patients with duodenal ulcer. In this connection, some obviously important problems remain unresolved. For example, if gastric juice is so corrosive, why do not the stomach and duodenum undergo continuous and progressive digestion? Why are ulcers usually so discrete and localized? The attempted solutions have always involved additional hypotheses and assumptions involving such concepts as defensive factors. These latter assumptions are unnecessary if gastric juice is not corrosive.

4.6. Bias

Many aspects of the etiologic analyses of ulcer disease involve serious biases of different types. For example, it has been pointed out that difficulties in measurement may obscure causal associations. The point is pertinent, since it is not yet known which facet of the secretion of gastric juice (if any) is relevant to ulcerogenesis. The study of gastric secretion in patients with duodenal ulcer is a most unsatisfactory example of the Berkson bias. Only patients with duodenal ulcers who present to doctors and, indeed, only patients who present to hospitals are usually studied.

Probably one of the most important types of bias involves the selection of control subjects, since these subjects (who are assumed to be normal) are never included in studies in accordance with acceptable selection methods but are always chosen at random from populations conveniently available to the investigator. Worse, control subjects are never endoscopically and prospectively confirmed as nonulcer patients.

4.7. Summary: Relationship between Putative Cause and Disease

If the putative cause is believed to be hypersecretion of gastric juice, the following would hold:

1. The prevalence of the disease is significantly higher in persons exposed to the putative cause than in those not so exposed.
2. Experimental reproduction of the disease (duodenal ulceration) occurs in higher incidence in animals exposed to the putative cause.
3. Elimination of the putative cause eliminates the disease.
4. However, if the putative cause is thought to be the secretion or presence of gastric juice per se, the prevalence of the disease is significantly

higher in persons exposed to the putative cause than in those not so exposed.

5. But exposure to the putative cause is *not* more common in patients with the disease than in control subjects.

6. One would *not* find a spectrum of host response, following exposure to the putative cause, with a biological gradient from mild to severe.

7. The disease cannot be experimentally reproduced in animals or human subjects.

8. However, elimination or modification of the putative cause eliminates the disease.

9. That the disease can disappear despite persistence of the putative cause.

10. Drugs can heal ulcers, although the putative cause is unaffected.

11. In neither case (gastric hypersecretion or gastric secretion per se) has a time (chronologic) order been established (i.e., it has not been shown that the putative cause precedes the ulcer disease).

5. ALTERNATIVE ETIOLOGIC BASES FOR DUODENAL ULCERATION

The very rapid changes in the incidence and prevalence of duodenal and gastric ulcers, and their prominent distribution in specific population cohorts, indicate the presence and changing levels of exposure to environmental ulcerogens. The occurrence of ulcers in certain persons either reflects individual susceptibility to the ulcerogen or indicates random involvement of the affected persons.

Two principal clinical characteristics of ulcer disease cannot be explained in terms of the secretion and etiologic involvement of gastric juice. First, the ulcers are usually single and focal and are often restricted during single and recurrent episodes of activity to the same area of mucosa. It is difficult to understand how ubiquitous intraluminal noxious agents (e.g., gastric juice) produce localized mucosal lesions, rather than inexorably progressive general mucosal disintegration. Similarly, because the duodenal bulb is, presumably, exposed to gastric juice during much of the day, it is difficult to understand why a considerable proportion of ulcers heal spontaneously and remain healed for long periods, despite similar amounts of acid and pepsin in the luminal contents during remission as during periods of active ulcer disease.

Second, whereas acute traumatic and chemical wounds of the mucosa of stomach and duodenum heal rapidly, ulcers are usually chronic and heal very slowly or, sometimes, not at all. Many studies have shown that gastric juice may temporarily delay, but does not prevent, healing of (experimental) ulcers. It seems, therefore, that one of the fundamental cause(s) of the ulcers is a failure of, or interference with, the normal healing of the mucosal wounds.

ANNOTATED BIBLIOGRAPHY

Baron JH: *Clinical Tests of Gastric Secretion.* Macmillan, London, 1978.

> This comprehensive monograph details the types and results of different secretory studies in controls and patients with ulcer disease.

Brooks FP: The pathophysiology of peptic ulcer disease. *Dig Dis Sci* **30:**15S–29S, 1985.

> An orthodox account of the pathophysiologic abnormalities recorded in patients with peptic ulcers.

Code CF: The role of gastric juice in the experimental production of peptic ulcer. *Surg Clin North Am* **23:**1091–1101, 1943.

> An early review of the subject, which has been very influential in forming current views of the topic.

Dragstedt LR: The pathogenesis of duodenal and gastric ulcers. *Am J Surg* **136:**286–301, 1978.

> An authoritative account of the experimental surgical procedures used to determine the relationship between gastric secretion and ulcer disease.

Feinstein AR: Clinical biostatistics. XLVII. Scientific standards vs. statistical associations and biologic logic in the analysis of causation. *Clin Pharmacol Ther* **25:**481–492, 1979.

> An excellent analysis of the relationships between association of two factors and their potential causal relationship.

Hunt RH, Howden CW, Jones DB, et al: The correlation between acid suppression and peptic ulcer healing. *Scand J Gastroenterol* **21:**(suppl)**125:**22–29, 1986.

> An example of the evidence linking therapeutic removal of gastric juice and ulcer healing.

Robert A: Experimental production of duodenal ulcers. *Biol Gastroenterol (Paris)* **7:**145–161, 1974.

> An excellent review of the different types of experimental approach used to produce duodenal ulcers in animals.

Sackett DL: Bias in analytic research. *J Chron Dis* **32:**51–63, 1979.

> An excellent account of the different sorts of bias encountered in selecting subjects for clinical studies.

Susser M: Rules of inference in epidemiology. *Regul Toxicol Pharmacol* **6:**116–128, 1986.

> A comprehensive account of the rules for inferring causality in an epidemiologic relationship.

Szabo S: Pathogenesis of duodenal ulcer disease. *Lab Invest* **51:**121–147, 1984.

> A comprehensive account of the etiologic inferences that can be obtained from modern animal experiments.

Wormsley KG: Duodenal ulcer: Does pathophysiology equal aetiology? *Gut* **24:**775–780, 1983.

> A critical review of the supposed pathophysiologic bases of duodenal ulceration.

Wormsley KG: Aetiology of ulcers. *Bailliere's* **2:**555–571, 1988.

> A comprehensive review of the possible etiologic bases of ulcer disease, assuming that gastric juice is irrelevant for ulcerogenesis.

3

Pathomorphology of Gastric Mucosal Injury

JERZY STACHURA

1. FUNCTIONAL MORPHOLOGY OF THE GASTRIC MUCOSA

Normal gastric mucosa shows regional differences. There are five regions: cardia, fundus, body (corpus), antrum, and pylorus (Fig. 1). The cardia that occupies a relatively small area at the esophagogastric junction contains mucoid glands with some acinar arrangement. The mucosa of the fundic area and body (corpus) of the stomach consists of oxyntic glands draining into gastric pits (Fig. 2). Oxyntic glands consist of parietal cells secreting acid and intrinsic factor, chief cells producing pepsinogens, and endocrine cells. The most common endocrine cells in oxyntic mucosa are enterochromaffin-like (ECl) cells and A (X) cells. Their hormonal products remain unknown. The antrum extends from the body of the stomach to the pylorus. The gastric mucosa in this region gradually (through the intermediate zone) converts into an antral type with mucoid glands containing mucus and endocrine cells, especially gastrin-producing G cells. The pylorus is the sphincteric orifice opening into the duodenum.

The gastric luminal surface is lined with surface mucus cells that also line the gastric pits. They are tall and columnar, and their apical portion is filled with mucus granules. They are able to secrete mucus into the gastric lumen. Mucus

JERZY STACHURA • Department of Cell Pathology, University Medical School, 31–531 Krakow, Poland; and Division of Gastroenterology, University of California–Irvine, Irvine, California 92717.

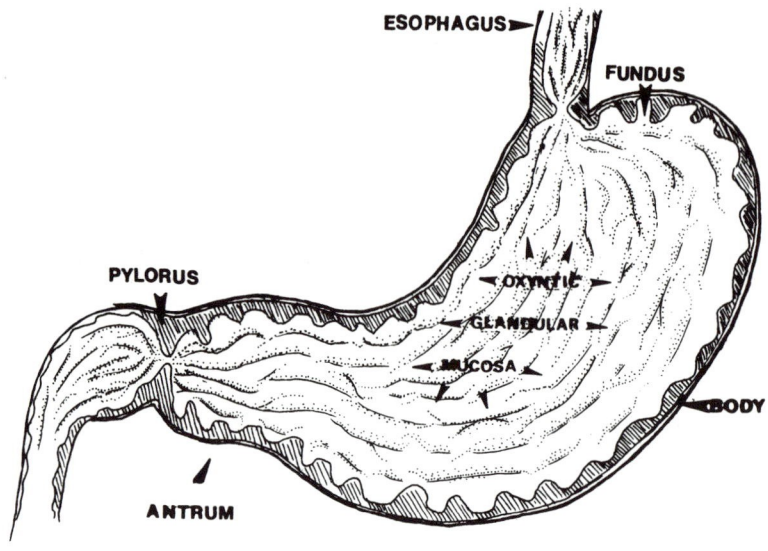

Figure 1. Anatomy of the human stomach.

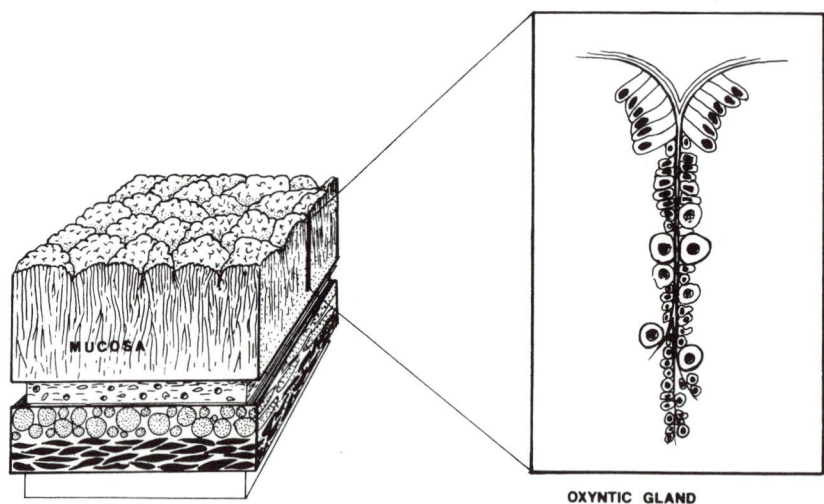

OXYNTIC GLAND

Figure 2. Histologic structure of the gastric oxyntic area. The mucosa is covered by surface epithelial cells. Neck cells, parietal (large, clear), and chief cells are located deeper below the surface.

together with phospholipids (derived from the membranes of surface mucus cells) form an unstirred layer maintaining a relatively neutral pH at the cell surface and protecting the gastric mucosa against digestion by gastric juice. Surface epithelial cells, which shed constantly at the rate of half a million cells per minute, are replaced by newly formed cells from the neck area. Usually it takes 2–3 days to replace the whole population of the surface epithelial cells completely.

Mucus neck cells cover the junction between gastric pits and gastric glands (glandular neck area). These cells resemble surface epithelial cells but have fewer mucus granules. In normal gastric mucosa, the glandular neck area constitutes a mucosal regenerative zone. Mucus neck cells are thought to be the progenitor cells for both surface epithelial and glandular cells. Glandular cells (parietal, chief, and endocrine cells) are characterized by a long life span (counted in weeks and months) and are usually lost by a process of apoptosis.

Parietal (oxyntic) cells produce HCl and intrinsic factor. The parietal cell contains numerous mitochondria that generate energy, tubulovesicles (a round or oval membranous structure), and canaliculi. During the unstimulated state, the tubulovesicles are numerous, while the secretory canaliculi are few. During secretory stimulation, tubulovesicles disappear and the secretory canaliculi become very prominent and elaborated. HCl is produced by H^+/K^+ ATP-ase exchanging H^+ for K^+ localized in the tubulovesicular and canalicular membranes.

Chief cells occupy the deepest portion of gastric oxyntic glands. Chief cells produce pepsinogens. The basal portion of the chief cell is composed of well-developed rough endoplasmic reticulum, while the supranuclear portion contains zymogen granules. Gastric glands are engulfed in the lamina propria, the connective tissue of the mucosa. The lamina propria contains numerous neural elements and very well developed microvasculature.

The muscularis mucosa separates the gastric mucosa from the submucosa, which is a connective tissue layer with very rich blood supply and neural elements (Meissner plexus). A thick and strong muscular layer (muscularis propria) and the serosa are the most external parts of the gastric wall.

Mucosal blood flow, vital for mucosal function, plays a crucial role in mucosal injury and most likely in mucosal protection. Mucosal blood flow depends on supply from submucosal vessels. Submucosal arteries divide into arterioles and these to precapillaries which penetrate the entire thickness of the mucosa as capillaries and bend just beneath surface epithelial cells and as collecting venules return to the submucosa. Several interconnecting capillary branches

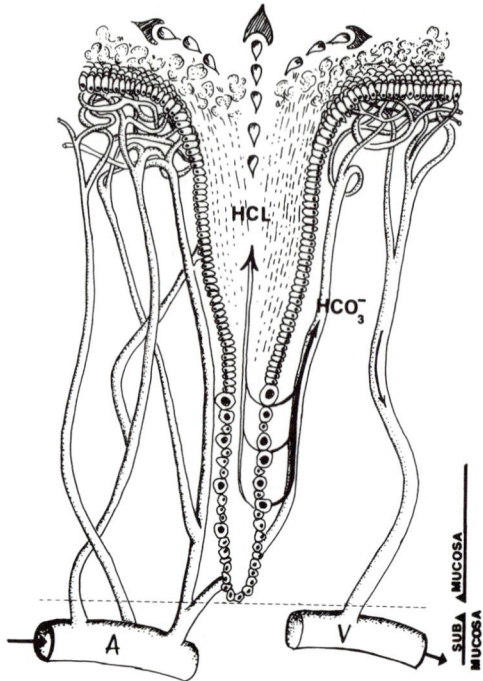

Figure 3. Structural relationship of parietal cells, hydrochloric acid, and bicarbonate secretion. Acid secreted by the luminal pole of the parietal cell is delivered into the gastric gland lumen, while bicarbonate is secreted by the parietal cells into the capillary and is delivered to the most superficial part of the mucosa, contributing to the formation of the alkaline microclimate.

are also present (Fig. 3). The capillary network closely surrounds oxyntic glands. While the glandular portion of the parietal cell secretes HCl into the lumen of the gastric gland at the vascular pole of the parietal cell, bicarbonate is released to capillaries and increases the buffering capacity of the mucosa at the luminal surface. Numerous arteriovenous anastomoses in the submucosa can redistribute blood flow in gastric mucosa and produce mucosal ischemia or congestion.

It has been shown that microvascular endothelium is a major target of acute gastric mucosal injury. Aggregation of platelets within injured microvessels leads to thrombi formation which impairs oxygen and nutrient transport and, thus, adds the ischemic factor to direct injury of glandular cells.

2. GENERAL CONSIDERATION OF CELL INJURY

The normal cell exists within a relatively narrow range of environmental conditions and structural changes. Within some limits, cells can adapt to alterations of the environment. Adaptation enables the cell to respond to physiological stimuli and to survive nonlethal injury. When the adaptive capabilities of the cell are overwhelmed, the cell sustains damage. This damage may be either sublethal (permitting recovery) or lethal (irreversible) (Table I). Despite its importance, our understanding of cell injury and death is still very limited. We do not know how much injury the cell can sustain, but histologic changes of irreversible cell injury and death become apparent within hours, while ultrastructural changes develop much earlier—some of them within minutes.

Steady-state kinetics and turnover of cell populations in tissues and organs are controlled by the process of apoptosis, an active process of cell self-destruction. Apoptosis permits a rapid and inconspicuous elimination of cells from the tissues. This type of cell death is often genetically programmed and is not associated with changes in membrane permeability. In the process, the cell rapidly condensates through digestion by lysosomal enzymes.

Necrosis or cell death, which occurs when injury becomes irreversible, is associated with changes in permeability of plasma membranes. Injured cells show deprivation of ATP, increased permeability, insufficiency of ion pumps, and deterioration of all vital functions. The morphologic counterparts of injury are swelling, and distortion of mitochondria, the appearance of flocculant densities in the cytoplasm, and clumping of cytoskeletal structures. Cell injury and necrosis are caused by hypoxia, physical injury, chemical injury, biological agents (infections), immune mechanisms, genetic defects, and nutritional imbalance.

Table I. Cell Injury: Toxic or Ischemic

Cellular signaling system overwhelmed
Cystolic calcium increased, activated protein kinases
ATP production decreased
Free radicals generated
Cytomembranes damaged
Sodium pump (ATP-dependent) impaired
Intracellular sodium increased
Cellular swelling, bleb formation—hypothetical point of no return
Cytoskeleton disrupted
Cell collapsed, necrotic

3. PATHOGENESIS OF REVERSIBLE AND IRREVERSIBLE CELL INJURIES

3.1. Ischemia

Aerobic respiration is primarily affected in hypoxia which results in depletion of energy sources (ATP), reduction in intracellular pH and Na/K$^+$ ATPase activity, sodium retention, and damage to cytomembranes as reflected by dilation of endoplasmic reticulum. Since the maintenance of low level of intracellular sodium is energy dependent, a decrease in ATP production results in increases in intracellular sodium, water accumulation and cellular edema.

3.2. Free Radicals

An increasing body of evidence suggests that free radicals are important factors in cell injury. Molecular oxygen contains two unpaired electrons in parallel spins. A free radical is any molecule that has an odd number of electrons. The intermediate products of oxygen metabolism are the highly active superoxide ion O_2, hydrogen peroxide H_2O_2, and the hydroxy radical OH^-:

Ischemia

$ATP \rightarrow AMP \rightarrow$ adenosine $\rightarrow$ inosine $\rightarrow$ hypoxanthine

$\leftarrow$ xanthine dehydrogenase

Reperfusion

xanthine $+ O_2 \rightarrow O_2 + H_2O_2 \xrightarrow{\text{iron}} HO^- + HO^- + O_2$

Free radicals can denature proteins by disrupting crosslinkages and are able to change cell permeability by causing peroxidation of unsaturated bonds in the fatty acids of membranes. All cells have antioxidant systems to deactivate free radicals. Superoxide dismutases, catalase, and the gluthione system are important in the deactivation of free radicals. Glutathione, a major source of sulfhydryl groups within the cell, is crucial in detoxifying hydrogen peroxide. In addition to intracellular antioxidants, living organisms benefit from extracellular antioxidants (ceruloplasmin, vitamin E, vitamin C, β-carotene).

3.3. Cellular Signaling System

Plasma membrane and cytomembranes are composed predominantly of lipids and proteins that form a discontinuous bimolecular layer of phospholipids and cholesterol, with globular proteins embedded within the lipid bilayer. The plasma membrane is the site for cellular receptors that form a complex signaling system. All cells try to adapt to information collected from their environment. Information comes from neural and hormonal signals as well as horizontal transmission from adjacent cells of the same organ. The attachment of specific molecules to receptors leads to activation of N protein. Activated N protein stimulates membrane-bound phospholipase C to cleave phosphatidylinositol-4,5-biphosphate into intracellular messengers, which activate protein kinase C and release calcium from intracellular storage sites. An increase in cytosolic calcium levels leads to cyclic adenosine monophosphate (cAMP) elevation and may activate calcium/calmodulin-dependent protein kinases.

There is a direct association between phosphatidylinositol turnover, diacylglycerol production, and arachidonic acid release from plasma membrane. Cell injury occurs when this signaling/messenger system is overwhelmed. At the point-of-no return, breaks in plasma membrane occur. Strong cytoprotective agents, such as prostaglandins, protect cells and tissues against injury but do not prevent the penetration of toxic agents (aspirin, alcohol) into cells and tissues. The most interesting area of the current research on cell injury is the inner leaflet of the plasma membrane, where the above-mentioned events take place and where the plasma membrane is in close contact with the cytoskeleton.

3.4. Cytoskeleton

The cytoskeleton is crucial not only for maintaining cell shape and structure but also for intracellular transport and cell adhesion to extracellular substrates. The cytoskeleton is a complex system of microtubules (relatively thick), thin actin filaments, and so-called intermediate filaments. Cytoskeletal proteins interact with a number of other proteins; for example, interaction with gelsolin results in conversion of cytosol from sol to gel. Microtubules are involved in bidirectional intracellular transport. Actin filaments take part in cell movement. Keratins are the major components of intermediate filaments in epithelial cells. Injured cells lose their microprojections or microvilli and change shape (round up). In severe injury, this is followed by blebs formation and eventually by cell collapse. Keratin filaments in necrotic epithelial cells are either disrupted and contracted or clumped in an irregular network surrounding a nucleus.

3.5. Calcium as Ultimate Cell Killer

Cytoskeletal function, cell signaling, and cell death are all calcium dependent. In a calcium-free medium, some cells, such as hepatocytes and neuroectodermal cells, are resistant to injury. Rapid calcium influx into injured cells appears to be a common final pathway that finally leads to cell necrosis. In irreversibly damaged cells, the rapid influx of calcium is not equalized by calcium sequestration in mitochondria and endoplasmic reticulum and/or by calcium extension to an extracellular space.

4. GASTRIC MUCOSAL INJURY

4.1. Acute Injury

The response of the gastric mucosa to injury is uniform regardless of the damaging agent; it usually results in exfoliation of the surface epithelium and injury of deeper mucosal layers. Deep mucosal injury is most likely caused, at least in part, by injury to the gastric mucosal microvasculature. Acute injury is most often produced by alcohol, aspirin, indomethacin, and other nonsteroidal-anti-inflammatory drugs (NSAID). Ultrastructural studies demonstrated that aspirin or alcohol cause damage in the endothelial cells of gastric microvessels as early as 1 min after administration. In most instances, acute gastric mucosal injury heals within several days.

4.2. Chronic Mucosal Injury—Acetic Acid-Induced Ulcers

A short exposure of rat gastric serosa to acetic acid results in gastric ulceration. Necrotic lesions of the mucosa are associated with vascular changes within the submucosa and the collecting venules of the mucosa. Acetic acid injury is a convenient model for ulcer-healing studies. Small acetic acid-induced ulcers heal within 2 weeks. Larger ulcers that rupture or penetrate the mucosa need much more time for healing. Four months after healing, the ulcer area remains abnormal both histologically and ultrastructurally. This abnormality could be the predisposing factor for ulcer recurrence.

4.3. Stress-Induced Ulcers

Stress can also be ulcerogenic. When rats are restrained and immersed in water, stress causes erosions and bleeding in the gastric mucosa. The necrotic mucosal areas are small or pinpoint in size but penetrate the entire thickness of the mucosa and bleed easily.

4.4. Endogenous Prostaglandins, Thromboxanes, Leukotrienes, and Platelet Activating Factor

It has been postulated that the increased susceptibility of the gastric mucosa to injury is associated with decreased generation of endogenous prostanoids, especially prostaglandin E (PGE). Drugs that inhibit the synthesis of endogenous prostaglandins, e.g., aspirin and indomethacin, are ulcerogenic. Immunization of rabbits with PGE induces gastrointestinal (GI) ulcers within 6 weeks. Passive immunization (passive transfer of PGE-hyperimmune plasma) induces gastric ulcers within 9 days. The segmental distribution of intestinal ulcers suggests that vascular involvement plays a role in ulcer formation.

Thromboxanes and leukotriene C_4, which are generated by conversion of arachidonic acid to unstable, but biologically very active products, lead to local mucosal vasoconstriction, causing ischemia and impairment of nutrient transport in the mucosa and increasing its susceptibility to injury. Leukotriene B_4 also a product of arachidonic acid metabolism is responsible for the chemoatraction of leukocytes and acute inflammation. Prostaglandins E_2 and $F_{2\alpha}$ (PGE$_2$ and PGF$_{2\alpha}$) are generated by the glandular cells (parietal, nonparietal, and macrophages), while leukotrienes are generated by polymorphonuclear leukocytes, vascular endothelium, and macrophages.

Platelet activating factor (PAF) is an endogenous phospholipid produced by many cells (e.g., polymorphonuclear leukocytes, macrophages, endothelial cells) and tissues. It has a potent biological effect, predominantly vasoconstriction, and is considered a proinflammatory mediator that interacts with other inflammatory mediators (histamine, leukotrienes, thromboxanes). It has been implicated in the acute gastric mucosal injury associated with endotoxin-induced shock. When given intravenously, PAF induces prolonged vasoconstriction and severe gastric mucosal damage.

5. PATHOGENESIS OF GASTRIC MUCOSAL INJURY

Gastric mucosa is continuously exposed to aggressive factors: acid, pepsin, and often bile acids refluxed from the duodenum (Fig. 4). The resistance of the gastric mucosa to injury depends on the function of unstirred mucus–bicarbonate layer, continuity of the surface epithelial cells, maintenance of blood supply, cell renewal, and neurohormonal regulation and adaptability of mucosal cells themselves. The importance of cell renewal and adaptability pertains not only to the

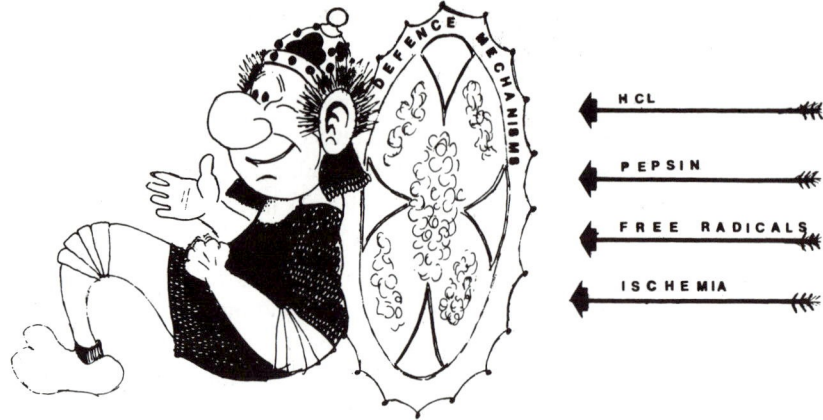

Figure 4. Diagrammatic presentation of mucosal aggressive versus defensive factors.

epithelial mucosal cells but also to the endothelial cells, which maintain the microcirculation. Numerous injurious agents cause exfoliation of the surface epithelial cells, which are rapidly replaced by cell migration. Strong irritants cause not only exfoliation of the surface epithelium but deep necrotic lesions that develop as a result of direct toxic cell injury, acid digestion of gastric mucosa, and blood flow disturbances. As a consequence of damage to microvessels, leakage of inflammatory mediators occurs and vasoconstriction of submucosal arteries results in ischemia. Reopening the constricted artery and perfusion of the ischemic area results in increased free radical formation and aggravation of the primary damage. The events leading to mucosal injury are summarized in Table II.

Table II. Gastric Mucosal Injury and Erosion
or Ulcer Formation

Direct toxic injury to surface epithelium, glandular cells, and lamina propria
Impairment of gastric mucosal barrier
Increased H^+ backdiffusion aggravating primary damage
Venoconstriction
Damage to microvessels, thrombi (in alcohol-induced injury)
Free radicals formation aggravated during reperfusion period
Discharge of proinflammatory agents (e.g., histamine, leukotrienes, fibrinopeptides)
Formation of necrosis
Exfoliation of necrotic mass
Erosions and/or ulcers

Inflammatory Changes in the Gastric Mucosa

Inflammation of the gastric mucosa may predispose it to injury and ulcer disease. Recently, *Campylobacter pyloris*—a spiral, gram-negative bacillus—has been rediscovered as a potential cause of chronic active antral gastritis. Endoscopic and histological examinations have shown that eradication of the bacillus brings normalization to the gastric antral mucosa and perhaps reduces the recurrence rate of ulcer disease.

6. RELEVANCE TO HUMAN PATHOLOGY

Most of the experimental data cited above are relevant to human pathology. Acute hemorrhagic or erosive gastritis is frequently associated with the chronic use of aspirin or NSAID, alcohol abuse, chemotherapy, uremia, severe stress, and shock. In acute hemorrhagic gastritis, the gastric mucosa bleeds diffusely from numerous erosions. Erosions are superficial lesions that are limited to the mucosa and that do not penetrate the submucosa. Histologic studies show that acute hemorrhagic gastritis is characterized by congestion, focal rupture of the mucosal microvessels, and the formation of hemorrhages and microscopic erosions, but not by acute inflammatory infiltration. Aspirin users or patients suffering from shock frequently suffer from acute ulcers or erosions, which are usually found in the antral area. These erosions or ulcerations are not usually accompanied by gastritis.

Chronic ulcer disease is a more complex entity. The pathogenesis of gastric ulcer disease relates mostly to decreased local resistance of the gastric mucosa rather than to the aggressive action of gastric juice. Disturbances in local blood flow and local ischemia are usually considered primary causes of decreased mucosal resistance. Chronic gastric ulcer shows morphologically deep mucosal and submucosal defects. Regenerating gastric glands are often present within the margins while the surrounding mucosa shows inflammatory infiltrates. The crater of the ulcer consists of a mixture of fibrinoid necrosis and granulation tissue. Granulation tissue usually penetrates the muscularis propria. Large submucosal arteries and veins are obliterated and occasionally show fibrinoid necrosis or vasculitis. Eroded vessels can be the source of bleeding. Another characteristic finding in the chronic gastric ulcer is markedly hypertrophied nerve bundles entrapped in scar tissue. Ulcer healing occurs when granulation and regeneration of epithelium predominate. The most recent data suggest that ulcers that appear to be healed by endoscopy remain histologically and ultrastructurally abnormal. These abnormalities may result in impairment of nutrient and oxygen transport and thereby be the basis for the propensity for ulcer recurrence. From this point of view, it is not the quantity (speed), but the quality, of healing that may be of crucial importance. This important issue of quality of ulcer healing should be addressed in future clinical studies.

ANNOTATED BIBLIOGRAPHY

Bendsten F, RosenKilde-Gram B, Tage-Jensen U, et al: Duodenal bulb acidity in patients with duodenal ulcer. *Gastroenterology* **93**:1263–1269, 1987.

This study indicates that higher delivery rate of acid into the duodenum found in duodenal ulcer patients is probably not an important factor in duodenal ulcer because efficient neutralization process keeps duodenal bulb pH within normal limits.

Ito S, Lacy ER: Morphology of rat gastric mucosal damage. Defense and restitution in the presence of luminal ethanol. *Gastroenterology* **88**:250–260, 1985.

This study described morphologic events taking place during ethanol-induced damage of the gastric mucosa and an early restitution of the surface epithelium.

Kitahara TK, Guth PH: Effect of aspirin plus hydrochloric acid on the gastric mucosal microcirculation. *Gastroenterology* **93**:810–817, 1987.

This experimental study indicates that aspirin-induced H^+-ion block diffusion causes formation of thrombi in the mucosal microvessels and constriction of submucosal arterioles; it is therefore the basis for mucosal damage.

Mergner WJ, Shamsuddin AM, Trump PF: Concepts of cell injury, in Harmon, J. (ed.): *Basic Mechanisms of Gastrointestinal Mucosal Cell Injury and Protection.* Baltimore, Wilkins & Williams, 1981, pp. 3–30.

This chapter describes sequential ultrastructural and biochemical changes in the cells during reversible and irreversible injury. Ischemic injury was given as an example.

Oates PJ, Hakkinen JP: Studies on the mechanism of ethanol-induced gastric damage in rats. *Gastroenterology* **94**:10–21, 1988.

This experimental study demonstrates the importance of the gastric mucosal vasculature and microvasculature in ethanol-induced injury.

Rasmussen H: The calcium messenger system. Parts 1 and 2. *N Engl J Med* **314**:1094–1101; 1164–1170, 1986.

These two papers discuss the importance of calcium in cell function specifically in receptor-mediated cell stimulation.

Redfern JS, Blair AJ, Lee E, et al: Gastrointestinal ulcer formation in rabbits immunized with prostaglandin E_2. *Gastroenterology* **93**:744–752, 1987.

This study showed that anti-prostaglandin antiserum produces ulcerations in the intestine and stomach. It stresses importance of endogenous prostaglandin for gastric mucosal defense.

Tarnawski A, Hollander D, Stachura J, et al: Prostaglandin protection of the gastric mucosa against alcohol injury. A dynamic time-related process. Role of the mucosal proliferative zone. *Gastroenterology* **88**:334–352, 1985.

This experimental study analyzed sequentially morphologic, ultrastructural, and functional changes in the gastric mucosa during ethanol-induced injury and prostaglandin-afforded protection. Pretreatment with prostaglandin protected the gastric mucosal proliferative zone against alcohol injury and in this way enabled restoration of the gastric mucosal integrity.

II

Defensive Mechanisms of the Stomach

4

Mechanisms of Mucosal Protection

SANDOR SZABO

1. INTRODUCTION

The analysis of mechanisms of mucosal protection cannot be separated from often referring to the pathogenesis of mucosal injury. Deductions from studies on the mechanisms of gastrointestinal (GI) mucosal damage are frequently applicable to the understanding of mucosal protection. One of the key aspects of these extrapolations is that, according to conclusions derived during the last decade of research on mucosal injury and protection, both processes seem to be multifactorial or pluricausal. Empirical studies and theoretical analyses performed during the nineteenth century and the early twentieth century generally centered on one damaging element, e.g., acid, pepsin, infection, ischemia. Consequently, protection was also postulated to be operational only against that single damaging agent. Therefore, the development and clinical use of specific protective drugs, such as antacids, antisecretory agents, and antibiotics. The recent popularity of infectious theory of origin of ulcer disease is actually the recurrence of cyclical trends (in intervals of about 15–20 years) following the first extensive implication by Virchow of apparent infectious agents in the etiology of gastric and duodenal ulcers. The consideration of those factors subsequently included bacteria, parasites, and viruses.

Most modern studies on the mechanisms of mucosal injury and protection have been performed on the stomach. It is therefore no coincidence that we know

SANDOR SZABO • Department of Pathology, Brigham & Women's Hospital, and Department of Pathology, Harvard Medical School, Boston, Massachusetts 02115.

more about damage to the gastric mucosa than we do about the duodenum and more about duodenal mucosa than about resistance in the small intestine. It is a logical expectation that most of the material and concepts presented in this chapter deal with the stomach, although relevant data concerning the duodenum, jejunum, and ileum are also cited.

First, concepts of cell and tissue protection should be distinguished; that is, with the introduction of the concept of gastric cytoprotection, emphasis focused on cell injury and protection, at the expense of neglecting the heterogeneity and complex structure of the gastric mucosa. The results were often disappointing and misleading and created unrealistic expectations among clinicians and drug designers in the pharmaceuticals industry. It is therefore appropriate to consider tissue or histoprotection and organoprotection while acknowledging that we are not entirely certain how certain cells are protected by specific agents, such as prostaglandins (PG) and sulfhydryls (SH), in the gastric mucosa. Furthermore, the initial protection does not need to be complete and perfect, yet tissue integrity is preserved and organ function more or less undisturbed. Last but not least, extramucosal components such as muscle spasm and blood flow also contribute to mucosal protection. Clearly, mechanisms of gastroprotection are indeed complex and multifactorial.

2. ANATOMICAL FEATURES OF GASTROPROTECTION

The mechanisms of protection in a complex organ such as the stomach are influenced by the local anatomical and histologic composition and structures. Gastroprotective agents may then affect one or several of these features while exerting their preventive or therapeutic influence. These interactions could be additive or potentiating.

It should be recalled that protection in the gut, as in most other organs having a moderate level of organization, may be achieved by at least two mechanisms: preserving the existing cells, or replacing the lost tissue (Table I). In the liver, for example, both processes are operational, while in the brain and heart, the highly specialized cells can barely migrate and do not proliferate; thus, the tissue defect in brain or heart is repaired by easily proliferating fibroblasts and other connective tissue elements.

2.1. Cell and Organelle Membrane Permeability

The action and access of exogenous or endogenous damaging agents are quite limited by the permeability of plasma membrane and that of individual

Table I. Components, Categories, and Mechanisms of Mucosal Protection[a]

Components and categories	Direct (D)/indirect (I) protection	Mechanisms
Preservation of existing cells		
Enhanced resistance	D	Increased level of antioxidants and scavengers
Decreased exposure (e.g., altered absorption, dilution, shortened exposure)	I	Proper blood flow, vascular permeability and motility, mucus, acid, and bicarbonate secretion
Replacement of lost tissue		
By original cells (e.g., epithelia)	I	Cell migration (restitution) and proliferation (regeneration)
By connective tissue (e.g., fibroblast, collagen)	I	Cell proliferation and production of extracellular matrix

[a]These categories and mechanisms are not inclusive; rather, they are illustrative with typical examples.

organelles. Damaging agents may either cross these membranes without causing extensive structural lesions or may actually lead to temporary or permanent morphological and functional membrane impairment. The intracellular accumulation of original damaging agents or their metabolites as well as endogenous mediators of injury (e.g., calcium, water) may then result in reversible or irreversible cellular damage.

Tight junctions and other intercellular barriers also control the passage of luminal damaging agents into the gastric mucosa and intestinal and submucosal spaces. Agents which would strengthen these intercellular junctions would restrict the spread of damaging hydrophilic agents in the GI tissue. Although the pathophysiological significance of these anatomically well-defined structures is established, effective protective agents other than a few experimental chemicals are not yet available.

2.2. Cell Migration (Restitution) and Division (Regeneration)

If the cell and tissue barriers are broken and cell death ensues, the necrotic cells may be replaced either by migration of surviving cells from the edge of the lesion (e.g., from gastric pits in the case of very superficial erosion in the stomach) or by division of surviving cells when the proliferating cells fill up the necrotic tissue.

The fastest means of repair of necrotic epithelium is by rapid restitution. If the lesion is very superficial in the mucosa and blood flow is maintained (see Section 2.3.), the reversibly damaged and healthy epithelial cells rapidly respond by expanding pseudopodia and migrating to cover the epithelial defect. The process is very efficient and, within 15–30 min, most of the damaged surface after intragastric (i.g.) ethanol administration in the rat is repaired by rapid restitution (Fig. 1).

Nevertheless, this effective protective mechanism is operational only under certain conditions. First, as this is an energy-requiring process, a well-oxygenated area with functioning microcirculation is essential. Second, related to the first condition, restitution is effective only if the lesion in the mucosa is superficial: deep necrosis causes cessation of blood flow in a relatively large area and basement membrane is also destroyed in addition to cell loss. The superficial nature of the lesion is achieved in animal experiments either by physical removal of the alcohol from the stomach (e.g., 30–60 sec, as was done in the initial studies on restitution) or by decreasing the penetration of damaging agents by barrier formation, dilution or other physicochemical processes induced by cytoprotective agents. Third, cells can efficiently migrate during restitution only if framework or scaffold is available, hence the additional importance of superficiality of lesions to preserve the epithelial or endothelial basement membrane.

Rapid restitution is thus an effective mode of repair, but it cannot be extensively and directly induced by cytoprotective agents. Some stimulation may be achieved *in vitro* in cell cultures if the energy source is ensured from the nutrient media. Restitution is rather an inherent property of the GI mucosa, and it may be naturally activated in the case of damage and if certain conditions are met.

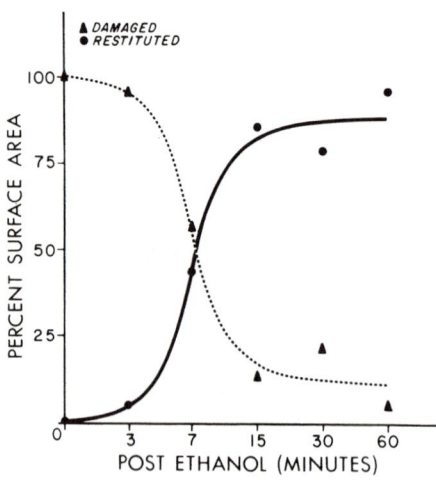

Figure 1. Epithelial restitution after short intragastric (i.g.) exposure to ethanol. "Damaged" indicates mean percentage of mucosal lengths with necrotic tissue attached to mucosa plus denuded basal lamina. "Restituted" stands for mucosal length with squamous-low cuboidal and columnar epithelium. (Reprinted with permission from Lacy and Ito, 1984.)

Dividing or proliferating cells contribute to mucosal repair irrespective of the extent of the initial lesion. Although this process also requires energy (hence blood flow), it can be directly stimulated by specific agents (e.g., growth factors). In the GI mucosa, most of the epithelial cells, unlike smooth muscle, proliferate readily. Fibroblasts also divide frequently, and the complex granulation tissue that fills up the deep erosion or ulcer actually consists of both young and mature fibroblasts, proliferating and expanding blood vessels, as well as chronic inflammatory cells (e.g., lymphocytes, plasma cells, and macrophages). The proliferating granulation tissue may become mature scar consisting of dense collagen and a few fibroblasts, which eventually may be covered by migrating and dividing epithelium (cf. reepithelialization). As cell proliferation requires some time (e.g., hours), this type of repair represents the latter event subsequent to rapid restitution.

Cell and tissue regeneration thus also represent important defense mechanisms in the GI tract and are operational under both acute and chronic conditions.

2.3. Microcirculation

Maintenance of blood flow is essential for virtually all the protective mechanisms of the GI tract. Although flow in larger vessels is also important, it is the mucosal microcirculation, because of its unique architecture and distribution, that is ubiquitously crucial for mucosal protection. Unfortunately, the vascular endothelium is also very sensitive to damage initiated not only by exogenous or luminal agents, e.g., HCl, pepsin, ethanol, aspirin, NaOH, but also by endogenous mediators, e.g., vasoactive monoamines, leukotrienes (LT), thromboxane (TX), and endothelin. Endothelial damage occurs early after i.g. administration of alcohol, aspirin, HCl, or NaOH and often precedes or parallels focal injury to superficial mucosal epithelial cells. Nevertheless, this microvascular damage, easily demonstrable by vascular tracers, always occurs before the appearance of hemorrhagic erosions. This is new but not surprising information; i.e., erythrocytes can escape only after substantial damage to the endothelium and vascular basement membrane.

Gastroprotective agents such as PG, SH derivatives, and sucralfate, which do not markedly alter the initial epithelial injury after i.g. administration of damaging agents, nevertheless diminish or prevent early microvascular lesions. This vasoprotection can be demonstrated both at the structural level (e.g., vascular tracers, light microscopy, and electron microscopy) and at the functional level (e.g., maintenance of blood flow). The essential part for mucosal protec-

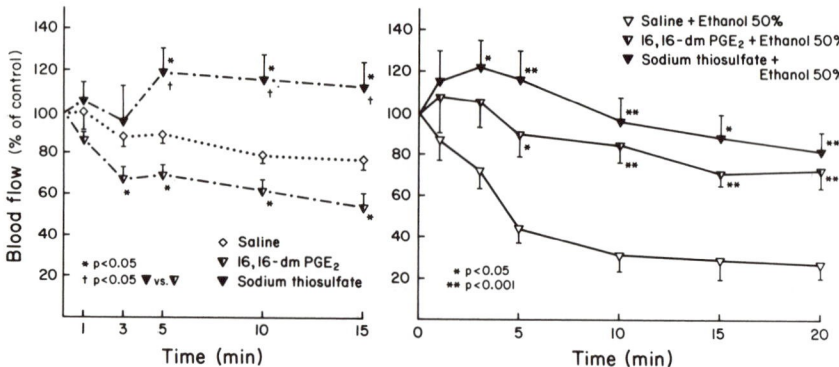

Figure 2. Gastric mucosal blood flow as measured by laser–Doppler velocimetry in the rat. The i.g. administration of 16,16-dimethyl PGE_2 or sodium thiosulfate was followed by either saline (left) or 1 ml of 50% ethanol (right). Although the protective agents alone (left) have different effects on blood flow per se, both maintain the mucosal perfusion at the control level even in the presence of alcohol (right). (From Pihan *et al.* 1986.)

tion is indeed the functional maintenance (not necessarily increase) of mucosal blood flow that permits the energy-requiring rapid restitution to repair the superficial epithelial damage. That is, gastroprotective PG and SH administered to normal rats usually have differential effects on mucosal blood flow (i.e., PG decrease while SH derivatives enhance microcirculation) (Fig. 2). After administration of ethanol, both agents maintain blood flow at the control level, indicating that their effect on blood flow per se does not count until a certain threshold. Rather, the protection against structural lesions in the microcirculation results in the maintenance of normal blood flow, even in the presence of damaging agents (Fig. 2).

If the mucosal lesions are severe, extensive, and rapidly developing, com-

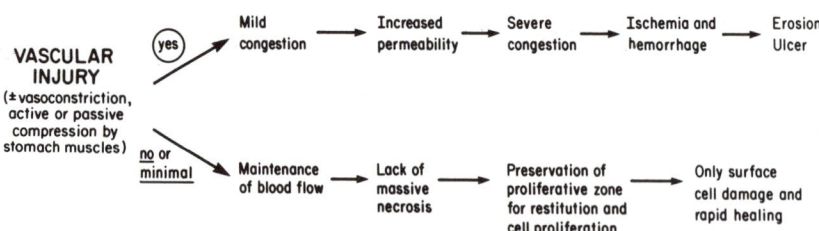

Figure 3. The importance of vascular injury in gastric mucosal injury and protection. (Modified from Szabo, 1987.)

plete microvasculatory standstill will preclude any substantial repair by restitution, leaving the cell proliferative process to replace the lost necrotic tissue. The latter process, however, takes hours to days, as opposed to just minutes required for restitution.

The status of microcirculation is thus central to the pathogenesis of mucosal injury (Fig. 3), as the extent of its damage is one of the determinants, whether deep anemic or hemorrhagic mucosal necrosis, or protection (i.e., repair with rapid restitution will ensue).

2.4. Muscle Tone

The tone and shape of the stomach are determined by the status of contraction and relaxation of the smooth muscle. Since the amount of muscular tissue is substantial, it is not surprising that the shape of the mucosa also depends on muscular factors. One theory implies that the nature of mucosal folds determines the linearity of hemorrhagic erosions after i.g. administration of concentrated alcohol, acid, and alkali. The dissolution of mucosal folds by PG apparently contributes to the gastroprotective effect of these agents; however, this remains controversial.

It has been known for some time that the rate of gastric emptying of acidic juice is a contributory factor in the pathogenesis of gastric and especially duodenal ulceration. Furthermore, motility, fluid transport, and the rate of the acid–base mix in the proximal duodenum are also pathogenetic elements in the mechanism of duodenal ulceration (Fig. 4). Pharmacologic modulation of gastric emptying, duodenal motility, and acid–base mix represent extramucosal mechanisms of mucosal protection.

The muscle tone in the stomach also influences blood flow to the mucosa. As in every organ that consists of mainly muscular tissue (e.g., cardiac and skeletal muscle), compression of thin-walled blood vessels is likely to alter blood flow. This probability is especially high in the stomach, where blood vessels cross the muscularis mucosae not only perpendicularly but obliquely as well. Emerging data indicate that smooth muscle contraction (e.g., in venules and the gastric wall), contributes not only to endothelial injury but to the rapidly developing congestion and stasis caused by ethanol. Furthermore, the development of hemorrhagic mucosal lesions seems to be limited to the area of congestion. Papaverine, which relaxes smooth muscle, prevents ethanol-induced hemorrhagic erosion. The tone of smooth muscle—either in blood vessels and/or the gastric wall—is thus an important factor both for the development and prevention of mucosal lesions.

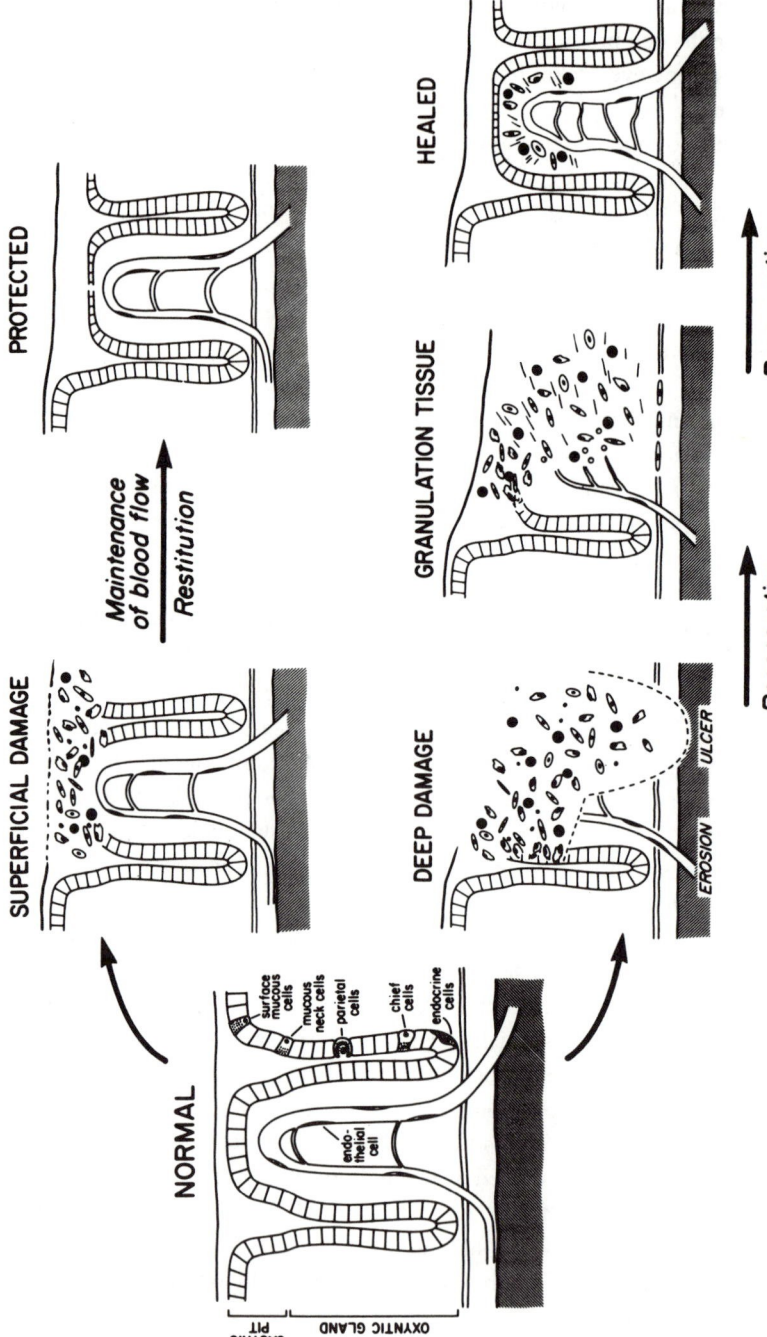

Figure 4. Normal, damaged, "protected," and healed gastric mucosa.

3. BIOCHEMICAL PROCESSES RELEVANT TO PROTECTION

Numerous biochemical and functional events may be involved in mucosal protection. Conceptually, however, at least two processes can be envisaged: enhanced resistance of mucosal cells or decreased exposure (e.g., diminished penetration, dilution, or shortened exposure) to damaging agents (see Table I). As the mechanisms of mucosal injury are multifactorial or pluricausal, it is likely that several processes are involved in mucosal protection. This does not mean, however, that all the components of protective mechanisms are equally important. It can easily be seen that one or two processes represent the major lines of resistance and that other processes provide only minor contributions (Fig. 5). Despite intensive research in several laboratories, the major determinants are suspected, but the major categories remain poorly defined.

a

Structural target

Vascular endothelium & basement membrane
Vascular & gastric smooth muscle
Mast cells & macrophages

Deep epithelial cells & neuroendocrine cells

Surface epithelium

Functional target

Cell and/or organelle permeability & contractility
Vasoactive products release
Cell migration (restitution)

Membrane transport

Membrane stabilization & tight junction

Blood flow
Muscle relaxation

Free radical scavenging
Mucus & bicarbonate secretion

"Mucosal barrier" stabilization

CELLULAR LEVEL

TISSUE LEVEL

b

Structural target

Surface epithelium
Vascularization
Deep epithelial & neuroendocrine cells
Mast cells & macrophage

Functional target

Mucus & bicarbonate secretion (↑)
Cell proliferation (regeneration)
"Mucosal barrier" stabilization
Acid secretion (↓)

Figure 5. Mechanisms of (a) acute versus (b) chronic gastric mucosal protection. The suggested mechanisms are categorized according to their likelihood of contributing to mucosal protection and healing. Boldface indicates major contributory role, italic indicates contributory role, and regular face indicates minor contributory role. (From Szabo and Pihan, 1987.)

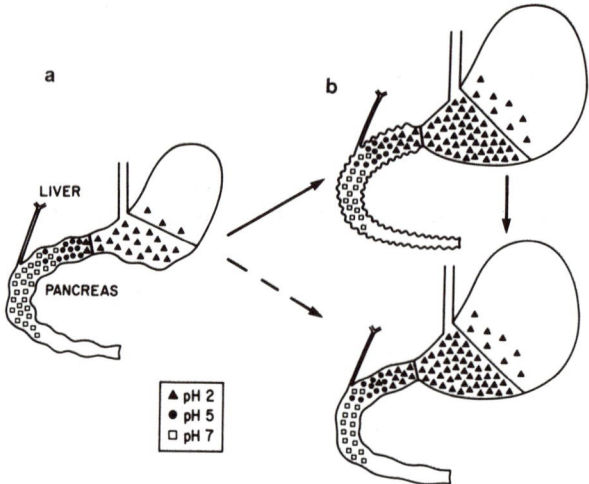

Figure 6. The acid–base mix in the proximal duodenum under (a) normal and (b) ulcerogenic conditions (displaced mix). (From Szabo, 1984.)

The importance of biochemical processes relevant to mucosal protection should also be evaluated as a function of time. That is, as gastric cytoprotection is an acute phenomenon related to prevention of acute hemorrhagic erosions without decreasing gastric acidity in most species, most of the processes reviewed here are relevant to acute protection (Fig. 5). For the chronic safeguarding of the gastric mucosa, mostly from acid pepsin injury, biochemical processes and functions different from acute protective processes seem relevant (Fig. 6).

Several biochemical processes relevant to mucosal protection are discussed in Section 3.1. The order of presentation does not imply priorities, which are, nevertheless, mentioned. The processes are listed as they occur from the luminal to abluminal sites in the stomach.

3.1. Mucus and Bicarbonate Secretion

The secretion of mucus and bicarbonate was one of the most frequently mentioned mechanisms likely to afford mucosal protection, a few years ago, especially around the emergence of the concept of cytoprotection. Intuitively, these are attractive explanations, especially because they postulate enhancement of the mucosal barrier (i.e., by the secreted and adherent mucus) and neutralization (i.e., of acid by the secreted bicarbonate). Gastric cytoprotection, however, is apparently an acid-independent phenomenon, so implicating bicarbonate as part of the mechanism is conceptually incorrect. Subsequent empirical work indeed proved that bicarbonate secretion plays a minor, if any, role in acute gastric mucosal protection against necrotizing agents (e.g., concentrated ethanol, HCl, NaOH).

The role of mucus in gastric cytoprotection is also more doubtful than was earlier believed. Studies are still being published with the faulty design and interpretation of results, e.g., that PG stimulate mucus secretion and that PG offer cytoprotection, leading to the incorrect conclusion that the major mechanism of mucosal protection is enhanced mucus secretion. Parallel occurrence of phenomena does not prove causal connection. This has been proved by a recent series of experiments showing lack of correlation between mucus thickness and mucosal protection by PG. Furthermore, drugs that solubilize mucus, such as the SH-containing reducing agents (e.g., N-acetylcysteine and mercaptoethanol), still offer dose-dependent protection against acute alcohol injury, although they may prolong healing in subacute and chronic damage. The SH-alkylator N-ethylmaleimide (NEM) injected subcutaneously abolishes gastric mucosal protection without influencing the release of soluble and adherent mucus, thereby dissociating gastroprotection from enhanced mucus secretion.

These results, however, do not diminish the crucial role of bicarbonate secretion in enhancing the resistance of gastric and duodenal mucosa to acid. Major breakthroughs in the elucidation of the mechanisms and source of luminally released bicarbonate occurred only during the past 10–15 years. We now know, for example, that bicarbonate is secreted mostly by the surface epithelial cells in the gastric mucosa, while in the duodenum it has at least three origins: absorptive cells of the mucosa, submucosal Brunner's glands, and pancreatic/biliary juice. The rate of bicarbonate secretion and its delivery through appropriate and coordinated gastroduodenal motility to the site of neutralization of acid (e.g., duodenal bulb) is one of the elements of protection against acid and acid-sensitive damage (see Fig. 6).

Soluble and adherent mucus (mucin, glycoproteins) released by specialized mucous cells in the stomach and goblet cells in the duodenum were also presented during the past few years as major defensive factors either against acid and/or pepsin. New data apparently indicate that although the mucus–bicarbonate barrier is effective defense against the penetration of HCl if the pH is 2.0 or higher (i.e., not very effective at high acidity), mucus seems to be a physicochemical barrier for pepsin. Phylogenetically, lubrication of gastric mucosa by mucus is also a natural defense against mechanical damage by rough food particles. A mixture of mucus and desquamated dead epithelial cells apparently may form a mucoid cap that provides a physical barrier against penetrating ethanol and acid.

Contrary to earlier interpretations, mucus and bicarbonate secretion is not a universal protective mechanism in the GI tract. Its role in creating a physicochemical barrier against mechanical irritation by food and water-soluble damaging agents, such as pepsin and acid, is undeniable. Mucus and bicarbonate, however, seem to add little, if any, directly to the acid-independent gastric cytoprotection, although they are essential components of chronic safeguarding of gastric mucosa against acid and pepsin. Indirectly, the mucoid cup seems to provide a barrier against luminal alcohol and acid. The fluid content of mucus and bicarbonate secretion may also contribute to the luminal dilution of damaging agents.

3.2. Hydrophobicity of Phospholipids

Phospholipids are the major components of surfactants, which keep most of the lung surface unwettable. Recently, it was extrapolated that similar molecules might exclude luminal fluid from the gastric mucosa. PG may increase the amount of these hydrophobic phospholipids in the stomach, while the degree of gastroprotection by milk derivatives is proportional to their phospholipid content. The relationship between luminal phospholipid and fluid may be more complex, however, than physical repellance. That is, ingestion of milk increases the resistance of lung despite the fact that milk does not come into direct contact with the lung. Biochemical incorporation of certain milk components seems the likely explanation.

Besides phospholipids, mucus glycoproteins have also been considered as biochemical fluid repellants. It is thus not clear at this stage whether the hydrophobic layer consists of phospholipids in the surface membranes of epithelial cells or rather that the extracellular mucus glycoproteins represent the hydrophobic film. In any case, these molecules may exclude or retard the absorption of water-soluble damaging agents, while they hardly influence the rapidly penetrating alcohols and other lipid-soluble chemicals.

3.3. Acid Secretion

Surprisingly, several lines of evidence indicate that a fully functional stomach with stimulated acid secretion is more resistant to damage than the organ at basal state of activity. The mechanisms of this enhanced resistance are mostly enigmatic, although a few clues are apparent.

The stomach with high secretory activity has enhanced blood flow; although it is not essential that it be increased for protection (cf. the importance of maintenance of microcirculation, discussed in Section 2.3), it may still help remove and/or dilute the penetrating damaging agents either through the bloodstream or through dilution in the lamina propria. The subepithelial capillaries also create an alkaline tide that helps neutralize hydrogen ions. Last, but not least, a secretory stomach is in high-energy status, which is also essential for many protective functions, including cell migration and restitution.

Since both pentagastrin and histamine decrease the extent of ethanol-induced acute gastric mucosal injury, it is likely that intraluminal dilution of alcohol by the secreted acid also contributes to this unexpected gastroprotection. It is also possible that dilution takes place within the tissue in a form of histodilutional barrier created by mildly increased vascular permeability and edema in the lamina propria after the administration of histamine (cf. Section 3.4).

3.4. Fluid Flux

Emerging data in several laboratories indicate that the rate of fluid flux and its accumulation in the mucosa (e.g., in the lamina propria) and in the gastric lumen also contribute to the mechanisms of mucosal protection. These results originate both from *in vitro* and *in vivo* studies. Experiments with isolated gastric mucosal cells and glands demonstrated that various cells in the gastric mucosa have different sensitivity toward toxic chemicals and that a relatively small change in the concentration of ethanol results in the preservation of most of the cells. After the vascular endothelium, parietal cells seem to be the most sensitive, with a very steep dose–response curve (e.g., the ethanol LD_{50} for cultured endothelial cells is about 6%, and 3–4% alcohol produces little or no damage). Very modest or no direct protection by PG or SH derivatives could be demonstrated with isolated or cultured cells; thus, the gastroprotection should originate chiefly from the dilution of toxic substances. Indeed, virtually all gastroprotective agents increase vascular and transepithelial fluid flux in the gastric mucosa. Careful histological examination of PG-treated control rat stomachs showed edema in the lamina propria. A histodilutional barrier created by slightly increased vascular permeability was proposed to contribute to the dilution of rapidly penetrating gastrotoxic agents, such as alcohol. Intraluminal dilution may also be a factor, although bulk dilution in the lumen is probably less efficient than dilution around the strategically important perivascular space in decreasing or minimizing vascular injury, in maintaining blood flow, and in ensuring the viability of the regenerating zone in the gastric pits crucial to mucosal repair.

Thus, enhanced fluid flux by gastric cytoprotective agents seems to contribute to mucosal protection by diluting the concentration of damaging agents either in the upper part of the gastric mucosa or in the lumen, or both. In addition, extravascular albumin and other plasma proteins may scavenge free radicals.

3.5. Free Radical Scavenging

Free radicals are potent mediators of cell and tissue damage in several organs, and there is some indication that they play a role in the development of gastric mucosal injury. The rapidly developing hemorrhagic erosions caused by concentrated alcohol, acid, and alkali are probably the result of direct chemical injury, while in lesions induced by aspirin, stress, or ischemia–reperfusion free radicals and lipid peroxidation may contribute to the development of mucosal lesions.

Prostaglandins are not known to scavenge free radicals, which, by contrast, readily react with SH compounds and with non-SH free radical scavengers as well as with specific enzymes (e.g., superoxide dismutase, catalase). Plasma proteins, especially albumin and ceruloplasmin, also scavenge free radicals; the presence of these proteins may represent one of the mechanisms of fluid fluxes, i.e., slightly increased vascular permeability associated with the action of gastroprotective agents.

3.6. Release and Action of Enzymes

One of the most investigated enzymes in the stomach is pepsin and its precursor pepsinogen. Although these enzymes have been implicated in the pathogenesis of chronic ulceration in the stomach and duodenum, there is little, if any, evidence for their role in causing the acute mucosal lesions. The release of lysosomal enzymes, however, has been implicated by some but not confirmed by other studies on the pathogenesis of acute erosions.

Proteases, especially thiol or cysteine proteases, released by cells or activated in the extracellular space have been implicated in gastric damage and protection by pharmacologic, biochemical, and histochemical studies. Ethanol-induced release of cathepsin B, a representative of thiol proteases, has been blocked by the SH alkylator iodoacetamide, which also prevents the development of hemorrhagic erosions. Interaction with these enzymatic proteins could thus be one of the explanations for the seemingly unusual gastroprotective effect of SH alkylators such as iodoacetamide and NEM administered i.g. in experimental animals. The regulation of release and/or the activity of available enzymes may indeed be one of the mechanisms of mucosal protection.

3.7. Release and Action of Vasoactive Substances

It is now well accepted that rapidly developing microvascular injury and stasis is a key element in the pathogenesis of acute mucosal lesions. The vascular damage is caused, in part, directly by exogenous chemicals, including alcohol, acid, alkali, and aspirin-like drugs, and by released endogenous vasoactive substances, including monoamines, LT, TX, platelet activating factor (PAF), and endothelin. These mediators usually increase vascular permeability in low doses (cf. histamine and bradykinin cause mucosal protection) but may produce endothelial damage and massively leaky vessels, which alone (e.g., PAF) may result in hemorrhagic erosions or predispose to the development of such lesions following i.g. administration of low doses of HCl or ethanol (e.g., after intra-arterial infusion of LTC_4 or LTD_4).

Balance in the release and activity of vasoactive substances is crucial to the integrity of gastroduodenal mucosa. Mice genetically deficient in mast cells showed significantly decreased hemorrhagic erosions after ethanol administration. Similar results were achieved in rats pretreated with histamine H_1-antagonists presumably by blocking the vascular actions of released histamine or fish oil extract, such as eicosapentaenoic acid (apparently by decreasing LT synthesis). Pharmacologic and dietary modulation of the release and activity of endogenous vasoactive substances is thus a recently recognized mechanism in the multifactorial approach to mucosal protection.

4. MECHANISMS OF ACTION OF MAJOR GROUPS OF PROTECTIVE AGENTS

The chemical compounds that decrease the severity of acute hemorrhagic or ischemic erosions without decreasing gastric acidity vary greatly in structure and pharmacological profile of action. In this diversity of structures and actions, no

Table II. Common Elements and Their Significance among Protective Mechanisms

Common elements and techniques	Contribution to gastroprotection
Direct cell protection	
Isolated cells	0/+
Cell cultures	0/+
Isolated glands	+/++
Indirect tissue protection	
Vascular integrity and blood flow	+++
Restitution and regeneration	++/+++
Intraluminal and/or histodilution	+/++

[a]Scale 0–3: 0, no evidence for significant protection; 1, minimal; 2, moderate; 3, major protective role.

structure–activity correlations have been recognized. Nevertheless, common elements with varying degrees of significance and contribution to gastroprotection can be easily listed (Table II).

Most of the compounds have been tested only in experimental animals, very few reaching human use in clinical tests. Accordingly, the mechanisms of action of gastroprotective agents is discussed by major chemical groups, and only clinically effective drugs are reviewed individually (Table III). The multifactorial nature of action of most of the gastroprotective agents is reaffirmed by the data presented in Table III. It is apparent that not one agent exerts only a single mechanism of action, although this does not imply that all the protective mechanisms are equally important for the group of compounds or individual drugs. The seven mechanisms of action displayed in Table III are not even complete, as they represent only the major categories studied extensively during the past few years.

4.1. Major Chemical Groups

4.1.1. Prostaglandins and Precursors

The naturally occurring compounds, prostaglandins and precursors, were the first to demonstrate gastric mucosal protection without decreasing gastric acidity in rodents. Despite numerous extensive studies, the mechanisms of their action are still poorly understood. A few candidates or mediators of their action, however, have been discarded as a result of intensive research work during the

Table III. Mechanisms of Action of Gastroprotective Agents[a]

Compounds	Vascular integrity	Blood flow	Restitution	Regeneration	Free radical scavenging	Mucus secretion	Bicarbonate secretion
Major chemical groups							
PG and precursors	+	+	+	?	−	+	+
LT antagonists and synthesis inhibitors	+	+	?	?	±	?	?
SH compounds	+	+	+	?	+	+	±
Non-SH antioxidants	?	?	+	?	+	?	?
Polyamines	−	?	?	+	?	?	?
Neuroendocrine factors	+	+	?	?	?	−	±
Metals	+	+	+	+	?	+	?
Individual drugs							
Sucralfate	+	+	+	+	?	+	+
Colloidal bismuth	+	?	+	+	?	+	?
Antacids	+	+	+	?	?	?	?

[a] +, effect; −, no effect; ?, not clarified or not tested.

past decade. Unsaturated fatty acids and other membrane lipid components may generate arachidonic acid, the synthetic precursor of PG.

Prostaglandins, like most gastroprotective agents, exert multiple actions, some or most of which contribute to achieve mucosal protection. Some of their actions are, however, paraphenomena and do not necessarily add to gastroprotection. For acute gastric mucosal protection, one of the most important actions seems to be the prevention of microvascular injury and maintenance of blood flow in the mucosa. This process ensures the availability of well-oxygenated blood in the upper mucosa and provides energy source for cell migration (rapid restitution) and subsequent cell proliferation (regeneration). It is also possible that PG exert some direct protection on the proliferative zone in gastric pits and/or individual cells in the gastric epithelium or vascular endothelium.

Most of the gastroprotective PG cause a mild increase in vascular permeability and stimulate the secretion of mucus and bicarbonate. This fluid flux— probably irrespective of its components such as mucin and bicarbonate ions— dilutes the damaging agents both in the tissue (e.g., lamina propria) and at the luminal interface. These actions seem also to contribute to the mechanism of mucosal protection by PG. An effect on smooth muscle tone might also contribute to gastroprotection, but there is only little or no evidence of direct protection of epithelial and endothelial cells by PG against damaging agents.

Although gastric cytoprotection is by definition an acute phenomenon, some processes elicited by PG and contributing to chronic safeguarding of the mucosa should be also briefly mentioned. Thus, although the rapidly developing hemorrhagic erosions caused by lipid-soluble (e.g., alcohols) and water-soluble chemicals are not markedly influenced by secreted mucus and bicarbonate, these endogenous chemicals are probably the first line of defense against the insidiously acting pepsin and HCl. Furthermore, cell proliferation (i.e., regeneration of epithelial and mesenchymal cells) as well as neurovascularization are more important in chronic than in acute protective mechanisms likely triggered by PG.

4.1.2. LT Antagonists and Synthesis Inhibitors

The major mechanism of action of LT antagonists and synthesis inhibitors is the inhibition of synthesis (e.g., by EPA and other dietary fatty acids) and/or antagonism of action of released LT derivatives in the stomach. Since LT are potent modulators of vascular permeability, these inhibitors and antagonists affect the microvascular changes. Through the vascular effects, needless to say, these compounds influence the development of acute erosions and ulcers. As mediators of inflammation, drugs that influence the synthesis and action of LT may also modulate acute and chronic inflammatory responses in the GI tract.

4.1.3. SH Compounds and Non-SH Antioxidants

SH compounds and non-SH antioxidants are endogenous (e.g., cysteine, methionine) and exogenous SH compounds (e.g., N-acetylcysteine, mercaptoethanol, dimercaprol) that exert multiple actions. From a mechanistic point of view, it is informative to know that the SH radical may be in reduced form or in various states of oxidation (e.g., -S-S-, -S-SO$_3$, -SO$_4$ as in disulfides, thiosulfates, and sulfates) to exert gastroprotection. This also implies that free radical scavenging, which is a unique action of SH compounds among gastroprotective agents, is probably not the most important protective action of these compounds. These implications are in agreement with the recent biochemical and pharmacological results. That is, there is little, if any, evidence of lipid peroxidation in the gastric mucosa during mucosal injury caused by chemicals and ischemia/reflow. Furthermore, relatively large doses of SH and non-SH antioxidants are needed to achieve gastroprotection when free radical scavenging probably plays only a small role in their mechanism of action.

The major mechanism of protective actions of SH compounds in the gastric mucosa is thus similar to that of PG, i.e., prevention or reduction of microvascular damage, maintenance of mucosal blood flow, and rapid epithelial restitution to repair the surface epithelial injury. Contributing factors might be a slightly increased vascular permeability, creating a histodilutional barrier and smooth muscle relaxation, ensuring proper outflow in the gastric microcirculation (i.e., removing the muscular component of microvascular stasis). A membrane stabilizing the effect of SH compounds should also be considered.

As with PG, there is little, if any, convincing evidence of direct cell protection by SH for isolated or cultured gastric cells. Gastroprotection by SH compounds may be attributable to indirect (e.g., vascular and muscular) effects and to the repair of superficial damage by restitution.

4.1.4. Polyamines

Polyamines are potent endogenous regulators of cell proliferation. Exogenous administration of spermine and putrescine, however, also prevents the alcohol-induced gastric erosions through an SH-sensitive process. Since cell proliferation is not a major protective mechanism against acute chemical damage in the gastric mucosa, it is likely that other actions of polyamines are relevant for this protection (e.g., influence on enzymes, membrane permeability).

4.1.5. Neuroendocrine Factors

Convincing evidence has accumulated from several laboratories that low doses of glucocorticoids, histamine, pentagastrin, and somatostatin offer gastroprotection. Very often, these are biphasic effects, i.e., low doses of steroids and histamine protect, while high doses cause or aggravate the gastric mucosal lesions. The protective mechanisms of these neuroendocrine products are poorly understood. Both glucocorticoids and histamine may slightly increase vascular permeability, creating a histodilutional barrier for gastrotoxic chemicals. Histamine and pentagastrin stimulate gastric acid secretion, which may also contribute to this dilutional effect. Glucocorticoids may also stabilize lysosomal membranes, potentially decreasing the release of hydrolytic and proteolytic enzymes. Somatostatin prevents ethanol-induced microvascular injury, as demonstrated by monastral blue. Our knowledge about the mechanisms of mucosal protection by hormones and neurotransmitters is thus very fragmentary, and we might be ignorant of the most important protective pathway(s).

4.1.6. Metals

Such metals as aluminum, magnesium, zinc, and copper prevent various forms of acute gastric mucosal injury through an SH-sensitive process that seems to be independent of gastric acid secretion and intraluminal pH. Since antacids contain metals, the recently discovered and unexpected gastroprotective action of antacids might at least in part be attributable to the effect of metals on gastric mucosa. Some metals (e.g., copper, zinc) oxidize or bind to crucial enzyme or membrane SH groups, influencing the activity of thiol proteases and membrane permeability, while others (e.g., zinc) accelerate wound healing. All the metals tested so far prevented the ethanol-induced microvascular injury and some stimulate mucus secretion.

4.2. Individual Drugs

4.2.1. Sucralfate

Sucralfate is probably the most widely used antiulcer drug that does not influence gastric acidity, yet prevents acute gastric erosions and accelerates the healing of chronic ulcers. The drug was introduced much before the recognition of the concept of gastric cytoprotection; nevertheless, it is not clear which of the multiple actions of sucralfate are the most relevant. Data exist that in experimental animals part or most of the gastroprotection by sucralfate is mediated by endogenous PG and SH. The drug also stimulates mucus and bicarbonate secretion, inhibits pepsin, and binds bile acids.

One of the most relevant acute protective actions of sucralfate and its active components seems to be the prevention of acute microvascular injury, maintenance of blood flow, and allowance of rapid restitution to repair the surface epithelial damage. Direct stimulation of mucosal proliferative zone to enhance mucosal restitution is also a possibility. For chronic safeguarding of mucosa, enhanced mucus and bicarbonate secretion, as well as antipeptic and bile acid-binding effects, seem to be the most relevant.

4.2.2. Colloidal Bismuth

Extensive clinical and experimental data with colloidal bismuth indicate that, like sucralfate, it prevents acute chemically induced hemorrhagic erosions and accelerates the healing of chronic ulcers. The relevant mechanisms studied thus far seem to include elevation of endogenous PG, interaction with endogenous SH, reduction of microvascular injury, and stimulation of mucus secretion.

4.2.3. Antacids

The acute gastroprotective effects of antacids have been shown to be independent of acid neutralization. This protection seems to be an SH-sensitive process mediated through the metal content of antacids. Further studies are needed to clarify this unexpected action of antacids.

5. SUMMARY

This review of the mechanisms of mucosal protection is focused on acute gastric and duodenal protection. It is emphasized that the discussion of mechanisms of protection cannot be separated from the analysis of pathogenesis of acute and chronic lesions in the stomach and duodenum. Thus, since the ulcerogenesis, by modern definition, is a multifactorial or pluricausal process, mucosal protection can also be achieved by multiple mechanisms, among which some actions of protective agents contribute more to gastroprotection than others. Conceptually, it is useful to categorize the components and mechanisms of gastroprotection and distinguish between (1) preservation of existing cells by either enhanced resistance of cells (e.g., by elevation of endogenous antioxidants) or decreased exposure to damaging agents (e.g., by altered absorption, dilution, shortened exposure), which can be achieved by the maintenance of proper blood flow, vascular permeability, motility, mucus, and bicarbonate secretion; and, if these mechanisms fail and tissue necrosis ensues, (2) replacement of lost tissue, achievable by either the original cells (e.g., epithelia) through cell migration (restitution) and proliferation (regeneration) or/and by connective tissue (e.g., fibroblasts, collagen) through cell proliferation and production of extracellular matrix. Among these elements, only the enhanced cellular resistance is identifiable as direct or true cell protection, while the other pathways represent indirect tissue protection. For acute acid-independent gastroprotection (cytoprotection), maintenance of blood flow in the upper mucosa and epithelial restitution are considered the key mechanisms of protection against the propagation of superficial lesions in the gastric mucosa. Dilution of damaging agents by fluid from microvasculature, secreted mucus, and bicarbonate also seems to contribute to acute mucosal protection. For the chronic safeguarding of the mucosa, proper mucus and bicarbonate secretion and gastroduodenal motility, as well as the ability to respond by cell proliferation are the proposed key mechanisms of mucosal defense. The molecular and biochemical aspects of protective mechanisms in the gastric and duodenal mucosa, however, require further and intensive investigation.

ANNOTATED BIBLIOGRAPHY

Bianchi Porro G (ed): DeNol: A new concept in cytoprotection. *Scand J Gastroenterol* **21**(suppl 122) :1–54, 1985.

Review of the new concept on cytoprotection, with special emphasis on colloidal bismuth (DeNol).

Brooks FP: The pathophysiology of peptic ulcer: An overview, in: Brooks FP, Cohen S, Soloway RD (eds): *Peptic Ulcer Disease,* Vol. 4. New York, Churchill Livingstone, 1985, p. 45.

This is a contemporary overview of the pathophysiology of gastric and duodenal ulcer disease. Although it focuses on the acid and peptic disorders, it covers other issues related to the pathogenesis of ulcer disease as well. It contains 700 references.

Derelanko MJ, Long JF: Influence of prednisolone on ethanol-induced gastric injury in the rat. *Dig Dis Sci* **27**:149–154, 1982.

The gastroprotective action of synthetic glucocorticoids is described.

Dupuy D, Szabo S: Protection by metals against ethanol-induced gastric mucosal injury in the rat. Comparative biochemical and pharmacologic studies implicate protein sulfhydryls. *Gastroenterology* **91**:966–974, 1986.

This paper describes the cytoprotective role of metals, with special emphasis on copper, zinc, and cadmium through an SH-sensitive process.

Flemström G, Turnberg LA: Gastroduodenal defense mechanism. *Clin Gastroenterol* **13**:327–354, 1984.

This review is concentrated on bicarbonate and mucus secretion, with special reference to the mucus–bicarbonate barrier. It briefly mentions some other protective mechanisms.

Guth PH, Poulsen G, Nagata H: Histologic and microcirculatory changes in alcohol-induced gastric lesions in the rat: Effect of prostaglandin cytoprotection. *Gastroenterology* **87**:1083–1090, 1984.

This microscopy paper documents the stages of congestion, as can be detected in histologic sections soon after administration of ethanol in the rat stomach.

Hawkey CJ, Rampton DS: Prostaglandins and the gastrointestinal mucosa: Are they important in its function, disease, or treatment? *Gastroenterology* **89**:1162–1188, 1985.

This is a major and very critical review of prostaglandins, summarizing the experimental basis and the clinical data so far achieved with cytoprotective and antisecretory doses of prostaglandins.

Hollander D, Tarnawski A, Ivey KJ, et al: Arachidonic acid protection of rat gastric mucosa against ethanol injury. *J Lab Clin Med* **100**:286–308, 1982.

This paper furnished evidence for gastric mucosal protection by the PG precursor arachidonic acid against alcohol injury.

Lacy ER, Ito S: Rapid epithelial restitution on the rat gastric mucosa after ethanol injury. *Lab Invest* **51**:573–583, 1984.

This paper details, for the first time, the importance of rapid restitution of cell migration, as well as the rapid healing of superficial lesions in the gastric mucosa.

Lange K, Peskar BA, Peskar BM: Stimulation of rat gastric mucosal leukotriene C_4 formation by ethanol and effect of gastric protective drugs, in: Samuelsson B, Paoletti R, Ramwell PW (eds): *Advances in Prostaglandin, Thromboxane and Leukotriene Research,* Vol. 17. New York, Raven, 1987, p. 299.

This chapter reviews the contributions of regulating leukotriene release to gastric mucosal injury and protection.

Leung FW, Robert A, Guth PH: Gastric mucosal blood flow in rats after administration of 16,16-dimethyl prostaglandin E_2 at a cytoprotective dose. *Gastroenterology* **88**:1948–1953, 1985.

This study describes that, in addition to histological evidence of congestion, functionally the blood flow decreases after ethanol, as measured by the hydrogen clearance technique and the flow is maintained if the rats are pretreated with prostaglandins.

Lichtenberger LM, Graziani LA, Dial EJ, et al: Role of surface-active phospholipids in gastric cytoprotection. *Science* **219**:1227–1229, 1983.

This paper describes the water-repellant properties of phospholipids and the modulation by prostaglandins.

Marks IN, Samloff IM (eds): Sucralfate in peptic ulcer and gastritis: A worldwide view. *Am J Med* **79** (suppl 2C):1–64, 1985.

This supplement summarizes the extensive data base on the experimental and clinical use of sucralfate exerting gastric cytoprotection and acceleration of ulcer healing in the stomach and duodenum.

Miller TA: Protective effects of prostaglandins against gastric mucosal damage: Current knowledge and proposed mechanism. *Am J Physiol* **245**:G601–G623, 1983.

This is an update on the rapidly developing field of gastric cytoprotection. Special emphasis is on the mechanism of action of prostaglandins.

Mizui T, Doteuchi M: Effects of polyamines on acidified ethanol-induced gastric lesions in rats. *Jpn J Pharmacol* **33**:939–945, 1983.

This excellent study demonstrates the gastric mucosal protection by polyamines.

Mózsik GY, Pihan G, Szabo S, et al: Free radicals, nonsulfhydryl antioxidants, drugs, and vitamins in acute gastric mucosal injury and protection, in: Szabo S, Mózsik GY (eds): *New Pharmacology of Ulcer Disease*. Elsevier, New York, 1987, p. 197.

This chapter reviews the role of non-SH free radical scavengers in gastric mucosal protection.

Pihan G, Majzoubi D, Haudenschild C, et al: Early microcirculatory stasis in acute gastric mucosal injury in the rat and prevention by 16,16-dimethyl prostaglandin E_2 or sodium thiosulfate. *Gastroenterology* **91**:1415–1426, 1986.

This paper describes the functional detection of congestion by the laser–Doppler technique. The ethanol-induced decrease in blood flow was counteracted both by prostaglandins and sulfhydryl derivatives despite the fact that these two protective agents, given alone, have differential effects on mucosal blood flow.

Robert A: Cytoprotection by prostaglandins. *Gastroenterology* **77**:761–767, 1979.

This editorial accompanies the first extensive experimental work and reviews the early data concerning gastric cytoprotection.

Robert A, Nezamis JB, Lancaster C, et al: Cytoprotection by prostaglandins in rats. Prevention of gastric necrosis produced by alcohol, HCl, NaOH, hypertonic NaCl and thermal injury. *Gastroenterology* **77**:433–443, 1979.

This is the first extensive experimental work published in a peer-reviewed journal on the concept of gastric cytoprotection.

Szabo S: Biology of disease. Pathogenesis of duodenal ulcer disease. *Lab Invest* **51**:121–147, 1984.

This review is focused on the pathogenesis on duodenal ulcer disease, with special reference to new developments in pathophysiology, such as the pathogenesis of preulcer lesions, correlation of biochemical and functional alterations, and pathogenetic elements other than acid and pepsin. It includes 335 references.

Szabo S: Peptides, sulfhydryls, and glucocorticoids in gastric mucosal defense: Coincidence or connection? *Gastroenterology* **87**:228–229, 1984.

This editorial succinctly summarizes the defense mechanisms of the gastrointestinal mucosa other than those related to prostaglandins (e.g., sulfhydryls, glucocorticoids).

Szabo S: Mechanisms of mucosal injury in the stomach and duodenum: Time-sequence analysis of morphologic functional, biochemical and histochemical studies. *Scand J Gastroenterol* **22** (suppl. 127):21–28, 1987.

This paper summarizes the functional and structural changes caused by ethanol and aspirin as well as duodenal ulcerogens, with special emphasis on the importance of vascular injury in gastric mucosal injury and protection.

Szabo S, Rogers C: Diet, ulcer disease, and fish oil. *Lancet* **1**:119, 1988.

This brief report summarizes the prevention of gastric mucosal injury induced by aspirin, ethanol, and other chemicals in animals pretreated with EPA to decrease production of leukotrienes.

Szabo S, Szelenyi I: Cytoprotection in gastrointestinal pharmacology. *Trends Pharmacol Sci* **8**:149–154, 1987.

This review is focused on the new interpretation of gastric cytoprotection in gastrointestinal pathophysiology and pharmacology. Emphasis is placed on the definitions and degrees of cell and tissue protection.

Szabo S, Trier JS: Pathogenesis of acute gastric mucosal injury: Sulfhydryls as a protector, adrenal cortex as a modulator, and vascular endothelium as a target, in Allen A, Flemström G, Garner A, et al (eds): *Mechanisms of Mucosal Protection in the Upper Gastrointestinal Tract.* New York, Raven, 1984, p. 287.

This brief paper summarizes the findings related to vascular injury in the pathogenesis of acute chemical-induced gastric erosions and endocrine factors in gastric mucosal protection.

Szabo S, Trier JS, Frankel PW: Sulfhydryl compounds may mediate gastric cytoprotection. *Science* 214:200–202, 1981.

This is the first demonstration that sulfhydryl-containing compounds exert gastromucosal protection and exogenous prostaglandin actions might be mediated in part by endogenous sulfhydryls.

Szabo S, Gallagher GT, Horner HC, et al: Role of the adrenal cortex in gastric mucosal protection by prostaglandins, sulfhydryls, and cimetidine in the rat. *Gastroenterology* 85:1384–1390, 1983.

This paper describes the permissive role of adrenal cortex, especially glucocorticoids in gastric mucosal injury and protection.

Szabo S, Trier JS, Brown A, et al: Early vascular injury and increased vascular permeability in gastric mucosal injury caused by ethanol in the rat. *Gastroenterology* 88:228–236, 1985.

This is the first paper in a peer-reviewed journal describing the rapidly developing vascular injury as revealed by vascular tracers, monastral blue, and colloidal carbon after administration of ethanol in the rat. The lesions were prevented by prostaglandins and sulfhydryl derivatives.

Szabo S, Pihan G, Dupuy D: The biochemical pharmacology of sulfhydryl compounds in gastric mucosal injury and protection, in: Szabo S, Mózsik GY (eds): *New Pharmacology of Ulcer Disease.* Elsevier, New York, 1987, p. 424.

This chapter reviews, in a book devoted to modern ulcer pharmacology, the role of sulfhydryls (free radical scavenging and other gastroprotective properties) as related to gastric mucosal protection.

Szelenyi I, Brune K: Possible role of sulfhydryls in mucosal protection by aluminum hydroxide. *Dig Dis Sci* 31:1207–1210, 1986.

This paper presents the SH-dependent action of antacids in cytoprotection.

Tarnawski A, Hollander D, Stachura J, et al: Prostaglandin protection of the gastric mucosa against alcohol injury—A dynamic time-related process. Role of the mucosal proliferative zone. *Gastroenterology* 88:334–352, 1985.

This paper compares the protective effect of prostaglandins and emphasizes the importance of the preserving of the proliferative zone for rapid restitution.

Tarnawski A, Brzozowski T, Sarfeh IJ, et al: Prostaglandin protection of human isolated gastric glands against indomethacin and ethanol injury. Evidence for direct cellular action of prostaglandin. *J Clin Invest* 81:1081–1089, 1988.

Important study demonstrating partial but statistically significant protection of isolated gastric glands against chemical injury.

Wallace JL, Morris GP, Krause EJ, et al: Reduction by cytoprotective agents of ethanol-induced damage to the rat gastric mucosa: A correlated morphological and physiological study. *Can J Physiol* 60:1686–1699, 1982.

This paper describes the importance of intact basal lamina as necessary to provide scaffolding for the migrating cells during rapid restitution.

5

Mucus Secretion

ADRIAN ALLEN, ANDREW C. HUNTER,
and ANWAR H. MALL

1. THE NATURE OF THE GASTRODUODENAL MUCUS BARRIER

Mucus is the major organic secretion of the gut produced by epithelia throughout the gastrointestinal (GI) tract. It is apparent as a viscous secretion slopping over the mucosal surfaces. In histological sections, the presecreted mucus endows the gastroduodenal epithelia with its characteristic neutral [periodic acid–Schiff (PAS) stain] and acidic (Alcian blue or high iron diamine) staining characteristics. Such observations do not, however, indicate the true nature of the protective mucus barrier, which is a layer of water-insoluble gel firmly adherent to the epithelial surfaces and forming a continuous protective barrier between them and the gastric juice in the lumen. It should be emphasized that this adherent mucus layer exists as a stable gel phase that is physically quite distinct from the viscous sloppy soluble mucus mixed with the gastroduodenal luminal contents.

A simple, direct method for observing the adherent mucus gel barrier is to view it by light microscopy on unfixed sections of fresh gastroduodenal mucosa. The mucosa, mounted luminal surface uppermost, is sectioned by a pair of parallel razor blades (1.6 mm apart). The physical stability of the adherent mucus gel is sufficient that it is not appreciably distorted by the sectioning procedure. Through-

ADRIAN ALLEN, ANDREW C. HUNTER, and ANWAR H. MALL • Department of Physiological Sciences, Medical School, University of Newcastle upon Tyne, Newcastle upon Tyne NE2 4HH, England.

out the operation, the mucosa and subsequent sections are bathed in physiological saline to prevent dehydration. The mucus barrier is seen as a translucent layer readily distinguishable from, and in between, the mucosa and luminal bathing solution. Adherent gastric and duodenal mucus is always observed as a continuous layer, but of variable thickness: 50–450 μm (medium 180 μm) on human antral mucosa, and 10–300 μm (median 80 μm) on rat gastric and duodenal mucosa. The mucus gel barrier can also be observed by a more indirect method using a slit lamp and pachymeter to measure gel thickness on an everted mucosa bathed with solution. The pachymeter is an image-splitting device that permits the measurement of optically distinct objects. Both methods for measuring the thickness of the adherent mucus layer give the same qualitative results, but the thickness dimensions from the pachymeter method are consistently about twice those from direct observation of unfixed sections. An explanation for this difference in thickness values between the two methods is that the pachymeter method is measuring a component of unstirred solution beyond the mucus gel surface, which remains on the washed mucosa.

For the adherent mucus gel to provide a fully effective barrier against gastric juice, its cover over the mucosa must be continuous. However, little if any extracellular mucus is apparent on a typical histologically fixed and stained gastroduodenal mucosal section; even when present, it is discontinuous. On the basis of such observations, some workers have questioned the existence of a continuous barrier over an undamaged mucosa. In support of their conclusions, the discontinuous network of mucus threads seen on electron micrographs of mucus is also cited. However, recent studies show that if the extracellular adherent mucus gel is first fixed *in situ* by such techniques as freeze substitution or with mucus antibodies, a continuous layer over the mucosal surface is seen on histological sections and electron micrographs. Further, and more importantly, a continuous adherent mucus layer is always seen on unfixed mucosal sections or on exposed mucosa by the pachymeter method. Evidence is now strongly in favor of a continuous adherent mucus barrier over the undamaged gastroduodenal mucosa.

An important feature of the adherent mucus barrier is its physical stability. Mucus gel does not dissolve when left in isotonic saline for 24 hr *in vitro*. Rheological studies on isolated mucus gel and studies *in vivo* demonstrate that its structure is unchanged following exposure to a wide range of pH values (pH 1–8), bile or hypertonic saline. Mucus gel is resistant to mechanical disruption but has the special characteristic of flowing over a relatively long period of time (about 1 hr) and of resealing when sectioned. Mucus gel also adheres strongly to cell surfaces. These properties facilitate the maintenance of a continuous and effective protective adherent mucus barrier over the mucosa.

Proteolytic enzymes (e.g., pepsin) will readily dissolve the adherent mucus gel by hydrolysis of the peptide backbone of the glycoprotein constituents that form the gel matrix. This has important implications *in vivo* in the stomach and, when the pH is low, in the duodenum. Thus, pepsin in the lumen will erode the mucus barrier to produce soluble degraded mucus glycoprotein. At the mucosal surface, a dynamic balance exists across the mucus barrier, where mucus lost at its luminal surface by peptic and mechanical erosion is counteracted by the secretion of new mucus. Since a continuous adherent layer of mucus gel is seen on the undamaged mucosa, it follows that normally mucus secretion successfully replenishes that lost by erosion. In cases of excess pepsin activity *in vivo,* however, this dynamic balance may swing in favor of peptic erosion, with resultant impairment of the gastroduodenal mucus barrier (see Section 4).

2. STRUCTURE OF MUCUS AND ITS MUCIN COMPONENTS

The principal gel-forming constituents of mucus secretions are high-molecular-weight (2 million or more) glycoproteins or mucins. Mixed within the mucus secretion are other GI secretions, such as enzymes and secretory IgA; microorganisms, sloughed off cells, and ingested food at various stages of digestion. Nonmucus components, both protein and lipid, have been implicated in determining the structure and functional properties of mucus secretions. However, a gel with the same physical structure and rheological properties as the native mucus barrier can be reproduced by concentration of the purified mucin alone. There is no reason to suggest that nonmucin protein or lipid components play an integral part in forming the gel structure.

The structure of mucins is very complex. However, sufficient is known to understand some of the structural features of mucins necessary for gel formation and the events leading to mucolysis. Mucins are composed of glycoprotein subunits ($5 \times 10^5\ M_r$) joined by disulfide bridges, to form high-molecular-weight polymers (having a molecular weight of millions). Each glycoprotein subunit consists of a central peptide core, with many closely packed carbohydrate side chains attached (Fig. 1). Each carbohydrate chain is composed of several sugar residues (up to 19 in length) in gastric mucus, and many will carry a negative charge because of the presence of ester sulfate and sialic acid residues. It is these negatively charged carbohydrate chains that give the mucin its acidic-

Carbohydrate side chains
(over 80% by weight of glycoprotein)

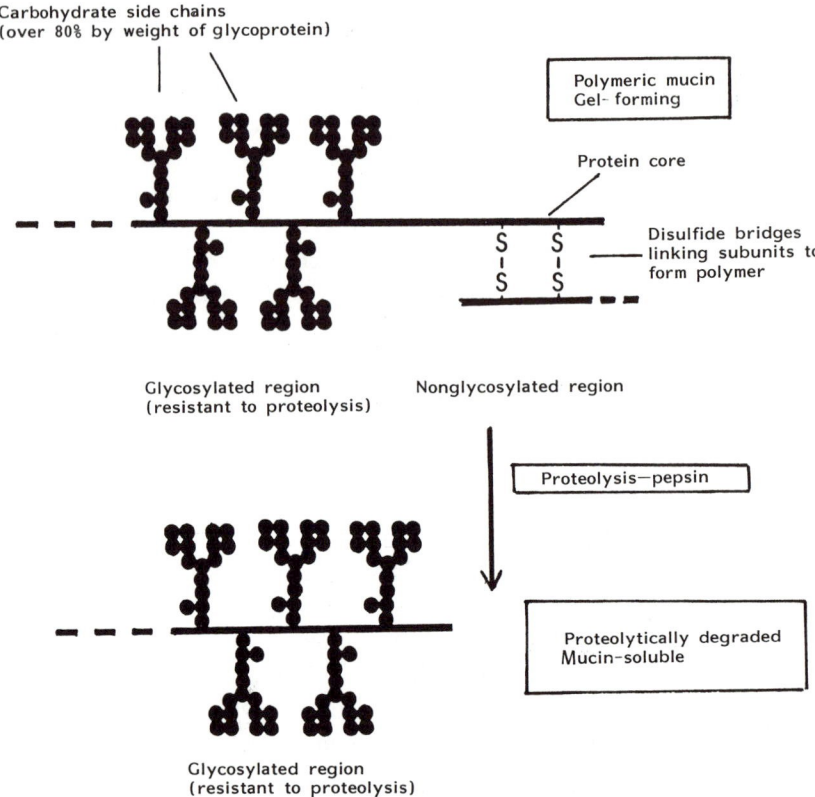

Polymeric mucin
Gel- forming

Protein core

Disulfide bridges
linking subunits to
form polymer

Glycosylated region
(resistant to proteolysis)

Nonglycosylated region

Proteolysis—pepsin

Proteolytically degraded
Mucin-soluble

Glycosylated region
(resistant to proteolysis)

Figure 1. Diagrammatic representation of gastric mucin structure. Pepsin digests the nonglycosylated protein core of the polymeric mucin to produce degraded mucin subunits. The polymeric mucin structure is essential for gel formation; the mucin subunits will not form a gel.

staining properties. Each glycoprotein subunit can be divided into two functional regions on the basis of the peptide core: (1) glycosylated regions in which carbohydrate chains form a closely packed sheath around the central peptide core, protecting it from proteolytic attack; and (2) other nonglycosylated regions of the peptide core that have little or no carbohydrate attached, which are therefore accessible to proteolytic attack by pepsin and other proteases. These nonglycosylated regions of the peptide core are also the site of the disulfide bridges that join the glycoprotein subunits together to form the polymeric mucin structure.

Gel formation between intact polymeric mucin molecules occurs at high concentrations, $\sim$50 mg/ml^{-1}, by noncovalent interactions. For gel formation to take place, the mucin must be in its polymeric form. This is the reason why proteolytic enzymes such as pepsin, which degrades the mucin polymeric structure, will dissolve mucus gels. Proteolysis digests the nonglycosylated regions of the peptide core, hence that part containing the disulfide bridges that join the glycoprotein subunits together. The resulting proteolytically degraded subunit consists of the glycosylated region, which is resistant to further proteolytic digestion. There is no detectable loss of carbohydrate during proteolysis and, since it is more than 80% by weight of the glycoprotein subunit, the proteolytically degraded glycoprotein is still quite large (approaching 5×10^5 M^r).

3. MUCUS AND PROTECTION AGAINST THE ENDOGENOUS AGGRESSORS

3.1. Acid

When considering the role of mucus in gastroduodenal mucosal protection, it is helpful to distinguish between (1) the natural endogenous aggressors, acid and pepsin, which are secreted in the gastric juice; and (2) exogenous damaging agents such as alcohol and nonsteroidal anti-inflammatory drugs (NSAID) not naturally occurring in the lumen and administered by man to himself or to experimental animals. Natural defense mechanisms have evolved against the natural aggressors, acid and pepsin. However, such mucosal defense systems may not be capable of resisting exogenous damaging agents, and the response of the mucosa, particularly to high concentrations of such agents as alcohol, may well be different. The adherent mucus gel covering the undamaged mucosa does not appear to function as an effective barrier against exogenous damaging agents such as alcohol. The primary protective functions of the adherent mucus gel, characteristic of the undamaged mucosa, are against the natural aggressors, acid and pepsin.

The role of gastroduodenal mucus in protection against acid is the provision, within the matrix of the mucus gel, of a stable unstirred layer at the surface of the mucosa. This unstirred layer in the mucus gel will remain despite the shear forces associated with the digestive processes. In such a stable unstirred layer, acid diffusing through the gel is neutralized by mucosal bicarbonate, with the establishment of a pH gradient from an acid environment in the lumen to a near-neutral pH at the mucosal surface (Fig. 2). If it were not for this unstirred mucus layer at the epithelial surface, the relatively small amount of mucosal bicarbonate would be rapidly mixed with the bulk of the luminal acid and no surface neu-

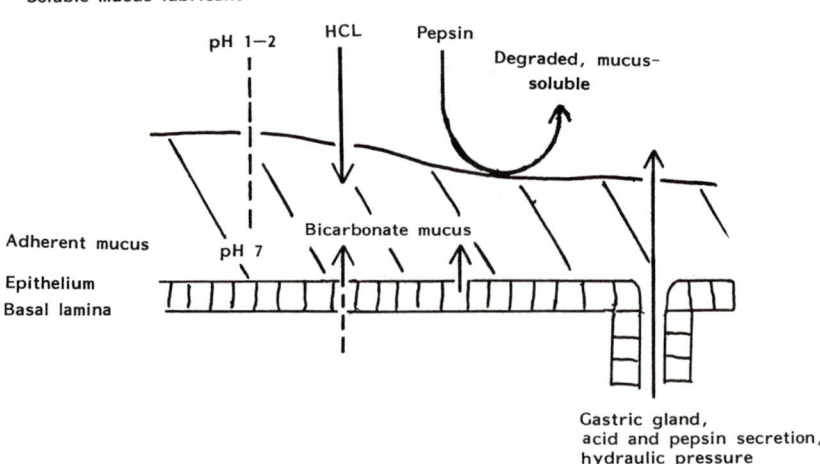

Figure 2. Mucus–bicarbonate barrier on the undamaged gastric mucosa, affording protection against endogenous aggressors, acid and pepsin. Adherent mucus produces a stable unstirred layer at the mucosal surface, to support neutralization of acid by bicarbonate. The mucus barrier prevents the diffusion of pepsin from the lumen to the underlying epithelium. (From Allen *et al.*, 1986.)

tralization or pH gradient established. The details of the role of mucosal bicarbonate in mucosal protection are fully discussed in Chapter 6 (*this volume*). It is important to stress, however, that the unstirred layer within the adherent mucus is stable under all conditions of acid pH that occur in the stomach or, for that matter, the duodenum.

While an integral part of the mucus–bicarbonate barrier to acid, the adherent mucus barrier is not a diffusion barrier to H^+ ions. The adherent mucus gel layer is 95% water by weight and is readily permeated by H^+ ions. These ions have been shown to pass through mucus gel at a rate approximately fourfold slower than their rate of diffusion through an equivalent unstirred layer of solution. Since H^+ ions diffuse very rapidly indeed through aqueous solution, even a fourfold retardation in this process will not significantly slow down their passage through the mucus gel. At such rates, acid in the lumen will equilibrate across the relatively thin mucus gel layer within a matter of minutes. Evidence for such conclusions comes from studies both on isolated mucus *in vitro* and on gastroduodenal mucosal permeability *in vivo* that demonstrate rapid H^+ permeability across the mucosa in the absence of sufficient neutralizing bicarbonate. Such observations also seem to exclude a meaningful role for lipid monolayers, which have been proposed by some to be an integral part of the mucus barrier to acid.

Furthermore, even when mixed with substantial amounts of mucosal tissue, mucus gel does not have significant buffering capacity compared with the large concentration of luminal acid.

3.2. Pepsin

The presence of acid in the gastroduodenal lumen is accepted as a prerequisite for the pathological process of peptic ulceration to occur. This is demonstrated by the therapeutic success of H_2-blockers. There is substantial evidence from experimental animal models, however, that the presence of pepsin per se can cause mucosal damage and ulceration. Several experiments have shown that while the gastric, duodenal, and jejunal mucosa are resistant to HCl perfusion at pH 1, the addition of pepsin to the infusate produces hemorrhagic lesions. Pepsin, but not acid alone, will induce acute esophagitis in rats; *in vitro*, it will cause a breakdown in mucosal resistance of frog gastric and esophageal mucosa. The progressive stages of pepsin-induced gastric damage can be studied by the instillation of pepsin into the pylorus-ligated stomach of an anesthetized rat. Instillation of acid pH 1 into the stomach alone for 1 hr does not cause observable damage to the adherent mucus or epithelium. However, the addition of pepsin (1–2 mg/ml) to the acid instillate results in a progressive disruption of the adherent mucus gel layer and the release of soluble degraded mucus glycoprotein over 2 hr. This is associated with the development of small focal hemorrhagic erosions in the epithelium and luminal bleeding. Such studies show that excess luminal pepsin (about two- to threefold above maximal) will progressively destroy the mucus barrier at its luminal surface at a rate faster than that at which it can be replaced by mucosal secretion. Once through the mucus barrier, pepsin is seen to readily digest the epithelium. There is indirect evidence for increased degradation of the adherent mucus barrier in humans *in vivo* following stimulation of pepsin. Thus, in gastric washouts from duodenal ulcer patients, there is an approximately threefold rise in both pepsin activity and soluble degraded luminal mucus glycoprotein following insulin stimulation. This increase in degraded glycoprotein is absent in vagotomized patients, in whom no increase in pepsin following insulin stimulation is observed.

The primary protective barrier preventing the pepsin in the lumen from normally digesting the surface gastroduodenal epithelia appears to be the adherent gastroduodenal mucus barrier, despite its progressive digestion by luminal pepsin. The matrix of gastroduodenal mucus gel is not permeable to high-molecular-weight proteins such as pepsins (32,000–40,000 M_r). Permeability studies show high-molecular-weight ions and molecules up to the size of at least vitamin B_{12} (1346 M_r) can penetrate the interstices of mucus gel but not, for example, the protein myoglobin (17,500 M_r). Therefore, the continuous layer of adherent mucus gel will provide a protective barrier to pepsin in the lumen by physically excluding its access to the underlying epithelium. Under normal circumstances, although pepsin in the lumen, together with mechanical forces, will erode the adherent surface mucus gel, new mucus secretion will maintain this protective barrier (see Fig. 2). It is only in special circumstances in which, for example, excessive pepsin digests the mucus barrier, as described in the pepsin damage model above, that the enzyme will gain access to the underlying epithelium and cause epithelial damage.

While the surface epithelium is sensitive to damage by both acid and pepsin, this cannot apply to the apical surfaces of the cells in the gastric glands, where there is no mucus–bicarbonate barrier. During secretion, acid at concentrations below pH 1 will be attained in the lumen of the gastric gland and here newly secreted pepsinogen will be rapidly and autocatalytically converted to pepsin. The apical membranes of the gland cells must be resistant to their own secretions. This has been demonstrated experimentally by the culture of monolayers of pepsinogen-secreting chief cells, which can adequately resist acidification of their apical surfaces to pH 2. Since a continuous cover of mucus gel is observed over the mouth of the gastric glands, the question arises as to how newly secreted acid and pepsin gain access to the lumen. A reasonable hypothesis is that the volume of acid and pepsin secretion creates a hydraulic pressure that physically pushes the secretion through the overlying mucus gel into the lumen. Current methods for observing adherent mucus would not show whether intermittent holes occur in the mucus gel cover over the entrance to the gastric glands during secretion.

4. IMPAIRMENT OF THE MUCUS BARRIER IN PEPTIC ULCER DISEASE

The protective efficacy of the adherent mucus barrier depends absolutely on its ability to form a gel—in peptic ulcer disease, this is deficient. Structural studies have shown that the polymeric structure of the component mucins is a prerequisite for gel formation. In fact, there is a direct correlation between the ratio of polymeric mucin to lower size subunit glycoprotein (or proteolytically degraded mucin) in the mucus secretion and its strength and overall stability measured by sophisticated rheological methods. The amount of polymeric mucin in adherent mucus from antral gastrectomy specimens can be measured by gel-filtration chromatography. This approach has shown that 67%, 50%, and 35% polymeric mucin is present in adherent antral mucus from control nonulcerated mucosa (removed for cancer of the pancreas), duodenal ulcer patients, and gastric ulcer patients, respectively. These groups were statistically different from one another, and, in fact, there was no overlap in the results for gastric ulcer patients and those from nonulcerated controls. Combining these data with those from structural studies on isolated mucus, it is clear that the adherent mucus barrier covering the mucosa of gastric ulcer, and, to a lesser extent, duodenal ulcer patients, is a weaker and poorer-quality gel than that covering nonulcerated mucosa. Further evidence for a disrupted adherent gastric mucus layer in peptic ulcer patients is apparent in unfixed sections of antral mucosa. Over the antrum from nonulcerated stomachs, a layer of translucent gel with a median thickness of 180 μm was observed, while that from gastric ulcer patients was markedly more heterogeneous and disrupted because of mixing of mucus with cellular material; although still continuous, accurate thickness readings were impossible.

Several possibilities might explain this breakdown in the structure of the adherent antral mucus in peptic ulcer patients. Evidence favors an increased rate of adherent mucus degradation, once it has been secreted, rather than a fault in initial secretory mechanisms themselves. At least three sources for an increased proteolytic degradation of mucus in peptic ulceration can be identified. First, it could arise from increased release of intracellular proteases (lysosomal) derived from necrotic cells, particularly because the rate of cell shedding is known to be higher in peptic ulceration. Another possibility is that it originates from *Campylobacter pylori,* a species of bacterium that is intimately associated with gastritic mucosa and recently shown to possess mucolytic activity. The third, and within the current context the most interesting, explanation is that it results from changes in the pattern of secreted pepsin types that are known to occur in peptic ulcer disease. Gastric juice contains different pepsins that can be separated from each other, on the basis of their charge, by electrophoresis. Pepsin 3 is the major pepsin in man, and pepsin 1 on average accounts for only 3.6% of total pepsin activity in nonulcer control subjects. However, in gastric and duodenal ulcer patients, pepsin 1 accounts on average for 23% and 16.5%, respectively, of the total pepsin activity present. What is particularly significant is that this ulcer-associated pepsin, pepsin 1, has been shown to digest mucus more readily than pepsin 3, both at the optimum pH 2.0 (twofold greater activity) and particularly at higher pH values (pH 4), where the difference is even more exaggerated (sixfold greater activity). Similarly, gastric juice from duodenal ulcer patients digests mucus more readily than that from nonsymptomatic controls both at the optimum pH of 2 and markedly at higher pH values (e.g., pH 4). Thus, the raised concentration of pepsin 1 in the gastric juice of peptic ulcer patients would be expected to result in an increased degradation of the adherent mucus barrier under conditions likely to prevail in the higher pH conditions of the duodenal bulb ($\geq$pH 4), as well as at the lower pH conditions of the stomach.

5. MUCUS AND PROTECTION AGAINST EXOGENOUS DAMAGING AGENTS

The mucus barrier is rapidly permeated by exogenous damaging agents, such as alcohol, NSAID, hypertonic saline, or bile salts, which are used in acute animal damage models. All these agents are sufficiently small in size to diffuse from the gastric lumen through the matrix of the mucus gel and, in the case of high ethanol concentrations, cause it to dehydrate in the process. The result is epithelial damage and exfoliation and, in more severe cases, vascular damage, hemorrhage, and visible lesions.

Following acute epithelial damage (except at the sites of haemorrhage), rapid repair occurs by the process of re-epithelialization (see Chapter 7, *this volume*). This process of re-epithelialization takes place in what must be a neutral and pepsin-free environment, achieved in two ways: (1) by plasma exudation, which provides neutralizing bicarbonate as well as washing the damaging agent away from the mucosal surface, and (2) following acute ethanol damage in the rat, by the formation of a thick gelatinous coat, often referred to as a mucoid coat, over the repairing epithelium (Fig. 3). This thick gelatinous coat is quite different in properties and composition from the original adherent mucus over the undamaged mucosa, although it has been wrongly designated as mucus by some. The gelatinous coat is substantially thicker (median 700 μm compared with 80 μm) and visibly more granular and sloppy in appearance than the adherent mucus layer. Histological studies using immunofluorescent stains for fibrin show this gelatinous coat to be composed principally of fibrin gel and necrotic cells, with the remains of the mucus gel as a relatively minor component. In the presence of this thick gelatinous coat, the re-epithelializing process has been shown to be protected against pepsin and from renewed alcohol insult. If the gelatinous coat is removed from the repairing epithelial surface (it can readily be removed mechanically with forceps), however, luminal pepsin or a further ethanol insult will prevent re-epithelialization. The formation of this protective gelatinous coat may be facilitated by the original adherent mucus gel, providing a template for the deposition of the fibrin gel. This is suggested by the effect of mucus gel on plasma coagulation times *in vitro*. In the presence of Ca^{2+},

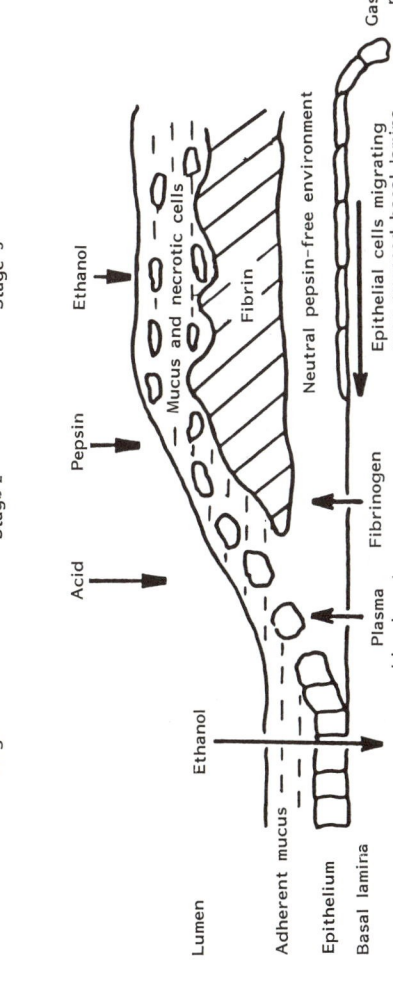

Figure 3. Ethanol damage and subsequent epithelial repair. Diagrammatic representation of formation of protective fibrin-based gelatinous coat. Stage 1: Ethanol penetrates the mucus barrier, causing exfoliation of epithelium and vascular damage. Stage 2: Plasma containing bicarbonate and fibrinogen flows out; note fibrin formation underneath remaining mucus and necrotic cells. Stage 3: Re-epithelialization protected from acid, pepsin, and now ethanol by fibrin-based gelatinous coat. (From Allen *et al.*, 1986.)

citrated plasma took 100 sec to clot, but this was virtually instantaneous in the presence of mucus. A fluffy gelatinous coat has also been observed covering the repairing epithelium following acute damage with hypertonic (1 M) saline, but it has yet to be shown whether this involves fibrin deposition.

6. MUCUS SECRETION, CYTOPROTECTION, PROSTAGLANDINS, AND OTHER ANTIULCER AGENTS

The protective efficacy of the adherent mucus gel barrier over the undamaged mucosa would be expected to be enhanced by an increase in its thickness. Median thickness of the mucus barrier has been shown to be increased up to threefold by neural stimulation (cholinergic), hormonal stimulation (secretin), and paracrine stimulation (prostaglandins). It should be emphasized that when assessing the protective capabilities of the protective mucus barrier, it is the adherent mucus gel layer that is the primary consideration. Many other agents have been assumed to stimulate mucus secretion by demonstrating increased output of soluble luminal mucus. However, soluble mucus has no obvious protective function against the gastric juice with which it is mixed. Further soluble mucus content in the lumen can arise by degradation of the adherent mucus gel as well as by direct secretion; it has been shown experimentally not to be an indicator of the thickness of the protective adherent mucus barrier. It is also important to make the distinction between intracellular mucin biosynthesis and the secretory process that forms the extracellular adherent mucus gel layer. Thus, the antiulcer agent carbenoxolone sodium has been shown to increase the rate of mucus biosynthesis, but it does not increase adherent mucus gel thickness.

An increase in the thickness of the adherent mucus layer, such as that induced by prostaglandins, would be expected to enhance protection against the endogenous natural aggressors, acid and pepsin. A thicker adherent mucus gel will provide a more extensive unstirred layer to support surface neutralization of acid. In protection against pepsin, the crucial factor would appear to be the maintenance of continuity of the mucus layer and therefore the thicker the mucus gel cover, the less likely it is to become discontinuous from erosion by peptic mucolysis or mechanical abrasion during the digestive process.

The cytoprotective effect of exogenous prostaglandins or endogenous eicosanoids (adaptive cytoprotection) in preventing deep-seated mucosal damage and hemorrhagic lesions appears to be mediated primarily at the level of the mucosal vasculature and is discussed fully elsewhere in this book. Damaging agents such as alcohol will still rapidly penetrate even a threefold prostaglandin-induced increase in the adherent mucus gel layer. A thickening of the adherent mucus gel barrier does not therefore play a significant role in the prostaglandin-mediated prevention of hemorrhagic mucosal damage. This is demonstrated experimentally by the observed lack of correlation between mucus thickness and conditions inducing cytoprotection. Protection against further ethanol insult can be provided by the mucoid cap formed following acute epithelial damage and subsequent repair. However, recent studies have shown that if this gelatinous coat is removed experimentally, prostaglandins will still exert their effect in preventing ethanol-induced, deep-seated hemorrhagic damage.

In designing suitable alternative peptic ulcer therapy to H_2-blockers, there is a need for good experimental ulcer animal models. Considerable attention has been given to understanding the ethanol damage model, the phenomenon of cytoprotection, and the process of re-epithelialization. In the ethanol model, adherent mucus appears to have at most a minor protective role; this is confined to its part in the formation of the mucoid cap of fibrin and necrotic cells covering the repairing epithelium. The pepsin damage model, while not yet studied in such detail, shows clear differences from the ethanol model. Thus, in the same animal model, only focal hemorrhagic epithelial erosions occur with pepsin, and not the total epithelial exfoliation followed by formation of the gelatinous coat characteristic of acute ethanol damage. The evidence suggests that the adherent mucus barrier does have a leading role in protection against pepsin and a strong supporting role in protection against acid.

ANNOTATED BIBLIOGRAPHY

Allen A: Structure and function of gastrointestinal mucus, in Johnson LR (ed): *Physiology of the Gastrointestinal Tract,* ed. 1. New York, Raven, 1981, pp. 617–639.

Detailed review of the structure and function of mucus secretions.

Allen A: Gastrointestinal mucus, in J.G. Forte (ed.): *Handbook of Physiology*—The Gastrointestinal System III. American Physiological Society, 1989.

A recent review on most aspects of mucus.

Allen A, Flemstrom G, Garner A, et al (eds): *Mechanism of Mucosal Protection in the Upper Gastrointestinal Tract.* New York, Raven, 1983.

This volume contains a large number of original articles by leading investigators in the field.

Allen A, Garner A: Gastric mucus and bicarbonate secretion and their possible role in mucosal protection. *Gut* **21**:249–262, 1980.

One of the first reviews on the mucus–bicarbonate barrier.

Allen A, Hutton DA, Leonard AJ, et al: The role of mucus in protection of the gastroduodenal mucosa. *Scand J Gastroenterol* **21**:71–77, 1986.

A short review summarizing current concepts of the role of mucus in mucosal protection.

Bell AE, Sellers LA, Allen A, et al: Properties of gastric and duodenal mucus: effect of proteolysis, disulfide reduction, bile, acid, ethanol and hypertonicity on mucus gel structure. *Gastroenterology* **88**:269–280, 1985.

The application of rheological methods to gastrointestinal mucus gels.

Bickel M, Kauffman GL: Gastric mucus gel thickness: effects of distension, 16,16-dimethyl prostaglandin E_2 and carbenoxolone. *Gastroenterology* **80**:770–775, 1981.

Mucus thickness measured by a slit lamp and pachymeter.

Filipe MI: Mucins in the human gastrointestinal epithelium: A review. *Invest Cell Pathol* **2**:195–216, 1979.

A useful review of mucus histopathology.

Flemstrom G: Gastric and duodenal mucosal bicarbonate secretion, in Johnson LR (ed): *Physiology of the Gastrointestinal Tract,* ed 2. New York, Raven, 1987, pp. 1011–1029.

An important review on mucosal bicarbonate secretion.

Flemstrom G, Kivilaakso E: Demonstration of a pH gradient at the luminal surface of rat duodenum in vivo and its dependence on mucosal alkaline secretion. *Gastroenterology* **84**:787–794, 1983.

Duodenal surface pH gradients.

Flemstrom G, Turnberg LA: Gastroduodenal defence mechanisms. *Clin Gastroenterol* **13**:327–355, 1984.

A short well-written general review on mucosal protection.

Harmon JW (ed): *Basic Mechanisms of Gastrointestinal Mucosal Cell Injury and Protection.* Baltimore, Wilkins & Williams, 1981.

A series of chapters on mucosal protection by leading workers in the field.

Ito S, Lacy ER: Morphology of rat gastric mucosal damage, defense, and restitution in the presence of luminal ethanol. *Gastroenterology* **88**:150–260, 1985.

An original paper on the salient features of re-epithelialization.

Kerss S, Allen A, Garner A: A simple method for measuring thickness of the mucus gel layer adherent to rat, frog and human gastric mucosa: Influence of feeding, prostaglandin, *N*-acetylcysteine and other agents. *Clin Sci* **63**:187–195, 1982.

The original paper describing measurement of mucus thickness on unfixed sections of mucosa.

Lacy ER: Gastric mucosal resistance to a repeated ethanol insult. *Scand J Gastroenterol* **20**:63–72, 1985.

A good review describing formation of the mucoid coat covering re-epithelializing mucosa.

Leonard A, Allen A: Gastric mucosal damage by pepsin. *Gut* **27**:A1236–A1237, 1986.

A short report on the pepsin damage model.

Morris GP, Harding RJ, Wallace JL: A functional model for extracellular gastric mucus in the rat. *Virchows Arch [Cell Pathol]* **46**:239–251, 1984.

A controversial view of the mucus barrier.

Morris GP, Wallace JL: The roles of ethanol and of acid in the production of gastric mucosal erosion in rats. *Virchows Arch [Cell Pathol]* **38**:23–38, 1981.

A key paper describing re-epithelialization and formation of mucoid coat following ethanol damage.

Neutra MR, Forstner JF: Gastrointestinal mucus: Synthesis, secretion, function, in Johnson LR (ed): *Physiology of the Gastrointestinal Tract,* ed. 2. New York, Raven, 1987, pp. 975–1009.

A comprehensive, well-written up-to-date review of the cell biology and structure of gastrointestinal mucus.

Pearson JP, Ward R, Allen A, et al: Mucus degradation by pepsin: comparison of mucolytic activity of human pepsin 1 and pepsin 3: Implications in peptic ulceration. *Gut* **27**:243–248, 1986.

The original paper on increased mucolytic activity of pepsin 1 in peptic ulceration.

Rathbone BJ, Wyatt JI, Heatley RV: Campylobacter pyloridis—A new factor in peptic ulcer disease? *Gut* **27**:635–641, 1986.

A short review summarizing current knowledge.

Robert A, Bottcher W, Golanska E, et al: Lack of correlation between mucus gel thickness and gastric cytoprotection in rats. *Gastroenterology* **86**:670–674, 1984.

An original paper showing changes in mucus thickness are not responsible for cytoprotection against ethanol damage.

Rozee KR, Cooper D, Lam K, et al: Microbial flora of the mouse ileium mucus layer and epithelial surface. *Appl Environ Microbiol* **43**:1451–1463, 1982.

An original paper showing continuity of the mucus layer under the electron microscope.

Sanders MJ, Ayalon A, Roll M, et al: The apical surface of canine chief cell monolayers resists H^+ back diffusion. *Nature (Lond)* **313**:82–84, 1985.

A paper demonstrating resistance of the apical cell surfaces of gastric glands to acid and pepsin.

Sellers LA, Allen A, Bennett MK: Formation of a fibrin based gelatinous coat over repairing rat gastric epithelium following acute ethanol damage: Interaction with adherent mucus. *Gut* **28**: 839–843, 1987.

The most recent studies on the mucoid coat, formed following acute ethanol damage, showing it is primarily fibrin and necrotic cells.

Sellers LA, Carroll NJH, Allen A: Misoprostil-induced increases in adherent gastric mucus thickness and luminal mucus output. *Dig Dis Sci* **31**:91S–95S, 1986.

An original paper showing prostaglandin-induced increased mucus thickness.

Silen W, Ito S: Mechanisms for rapid re-epithelialization of the gastric mucosal surface. *Annu Rev Physiol* **47**:217–229, 1985.

A good review on re-epithelialization and formation of mucoid coat.

Taylor WH: Biochemistry and pathological physiology of pepsin 1. *Adv Clin Enzymol* **2**:79–81, 1982.

A review of pepsins in gastric juice.

Wallace JL: Increased resistance of the rat gastric mucosa to hemorrhagic damage after exposure to an irritant. *Gastroenterology* **94**:22–32, 1988.

An original paper showing protection against hemorrhagic lesions in the absence of the mucoid coat.

Wallace JL, Whittle BJR: Role of mucus in the repair of gastric epithelial damage in the rat. Inhibition of epithelial recovery by mucolytic agents. *Gastroenterology* **91**:603–611, 1986.

An interesting paper on the mucoid coat.

Williams SE, Turnberg LA: Retardation of acid diffusion by pig gastric mucus: A potential role in mucosal protection. *Gastroenterology* **79**:299–304, 1980.

An example of studies on H^+ diffusion through mucus.

Williams SE, Turnberg LA: Studies of the "protective" properties of gastric mucus: Evidence for a mucus-bicarbonate barrier. *Gut* **22**:94–96, 1981.

The original paper on the pH gradient at the gastric mucosal surface.

Younan F, Pearson JP, Allen A, et al: Changes in the structure of the mucous gel on the mucosal surface of the stomach in association with peptic ulcer disease. *Gastroenterology* **82**:827–831, 1982.

The original paper showing a breakdown in mucus polymeric structure in peptic ulcer disease.

6

Bicarbonate Secretion and the Alkaline Microclimate

CHRISTOPHER J. SHORROCK and WYNNE D. W. REES

1. INTRODUCTION

The surface mucosa of the healthy stomach and duodenum is continually exposed to a corrosive mixture of hydrochloric acid, pepsin, transient reflux of bile (exposing the stomach to the detergent effects of bile salts), food with varied consistency and temperature, microorganisms, and in some instances alcohol and drugs. In the duodenum, acid emptying from the stomach is rapidly neutralized, but pH values of ~2 may still occur in the proximal duodenum for variable lengths of time. Clearly, these aggressive damaging luminal factors, along with ingested agents such as nonsteroidal anti-inflammatory drugs (NSAID) and alcohol, must be balanced by defense and repair processes, if mucosal integrity is to be maintained.

The concept of mucosal defense has come a long way since the work of Pavlov (1898) and Florey (1939), who performed important experiments on the ability of the duodenum to resist acid and pepsin. A number of factors have now been identified as being important in mucosal resistance to acid and pepsin (Fig. 1). The first line of defense is the thick layer of adherent mucus gel that covers gastric and duodenal mucosa. This was thought to contribute very little to overall gastroduodenal defense, until the demonstration of alkali secretion into

---

CHRISTOPHER J. SHORROCK and WYNNE D. W. REES • Department of Gastroenterology, Hope Hospital, University of Manchester School of Medicine, Salford M6 8HD, England.

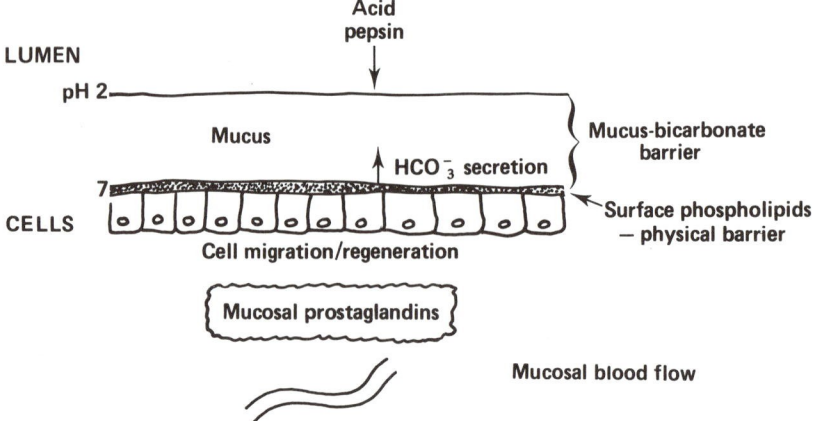

Figure 1. Diagrammatic representation of the possible components of gastroduodenal mucosal defense.

the mucus layer from underlying epithelial cells by Flemstrom (1977). This mucus-bicarbonate barrier sustains a pH gradient between the lumen and cell surface such that epithelial cells are maintained at pH 7–8 despite the presence of intraluminal acid. The epithelial cells form a second line of defense and, since the pH gradient may be overwhelmed by the physiological concentrations of intraluminal acid, this mechanism may be important in maintaining mucosal integrity. The physical barrier properties of the gastric apical cell membrane and intercellular junctions, together with the presence of surface active phospholipids on the membrane, may be responsible for preventing hydrogen ions from diffusing into the mucosa. Furthermore, epithelial cells are capable of rapid turnover and migration and may cover a defect in the epithelium within a few hours. The aftermath of mucosal damage may generate a further defense mechanism, a thick layer of mucus containing sloughed epithelial cells, together with passive movement of bicarbonate-rich fluid from damaged mucosa. This may prevent exposure of undamaged cell nests to acid and thus aid re-epithelialization. Finally, mucosal blood flow plays a vital role in maintaining epithelial integrity; studies have shown that increasing or decreasing mucosal blood flow will reduce or enhance susceptibility to damage, respectively. Blood flow, in addition to delivering oxygen and essential nutrients to the cells, also supplies bicarbonate; it may also remove diffused hydrogen ions.

2. BICARBONATE SECRETION

2.1. Historical Background

The existence of gastric bicarbonate secretion was suggested as early as 1892 by the Danish physiologist Schierbeck. In a series of carefully conducted controlled experiments in dogs, Schierbeck showed that feeding increased not only acid secretion but the amount of luminal CO_2 as well. These CO_2 levels (>100 mm Hg) were considerably greater than the levels in blood, reflecting gastric intraluminal interaction between H^+ and HCO_3^-. Thus, almost a century ago, there was evidence for the existence of gastric bicarbonate secretion. Shortly afterward in 1898, Pavlov suggested that alkaline mucus-lined gastric mucosa neutralizing luminal acid. Because of the magnitude of this secretion, it was dismissed as providing little contribution to mucosal defense. Little new work arose in this area until 1939, when Florey and co-workers demonstrated that the duodenum is much better at resisting instillation of gastric juice than is the distal small bowel. In the absence of pancreatobiliary secretion, this acid resistance of the duodenum was attributed to neutralization by bicarbonate secretion from Brunner glands or from the mucosa itself. The occurrence of gastric bicarbonate secretion was demonstrated by Grossman (1959), who studied antral pouches, and by Hollander (1954) in fundic pouches, after inhibition of H^+ secretion by vagotomy and antrectomy. Heatley (1959) suggested that protection of the gastric epithelium from acid could be afforded by bicarbonate transport from mucosa into the adherent mucus gel layer. This would provide a zone of low turbulence, supporting a pH gradient generated by acid–bicarbonate interaction. At this time, a pH gradient could not be demonstrated experimentally, and the hypothesis became superseded by the mucosal barrier hypothesis proposed by Code and Davenport (1964). These investigators considered that a gastric mucosal barrier, formed by the apical membrane of surface cells together with the tight junctions linking adjacent cells, was responsible for the low permeability of the mucosa to ions. A major problem in attempting to measure gastric bicarbonate secretion was the simultaneous and much greater secretion of hydrogen ions. Not until the development of potent inhibitors of gastric acid secretion did it become feasible to measure gastric bicarbonate secretion. The gastric juice of patients with achlorhydria as well as that of normal subjects was known to contain bicarbonate, but pioneering work by Flemstrom (1977) proved the existence of bicarbonate secretion from fundic and antral mucosa by a metabolically dependent process as well as by passive diffusion. His findings have subsequently been corroborated by other workers, and gastroduodenal bicarbonate secretion has now been documented in a large number of experimental models, including the intact human stomach and proximal duodenum.

2.2. Measurement of Bicarbonate Secretion

2.2.1. In Vitro

Antral or fundic mucosa stripped of muscularis externa from amphibian, rabbit, guinea pig, canine, and porcine stomachs have been mounted as a membrane in modified Ussing chambers (Fig. 2). This technique permits control of the environment on both sides of the epithelium as well as the study of some electrical properties of the mucosa. Antral mucosa contains no acid-secreting cells and spontaneously secretes alkali, whereas the acid secretion of the fundic mucosa is inhibited, usually by means of H_2-receptor antagonists.

Duodenal bicarbonate secretion is similarly measured, except that the tissue may be mounted as a cylinder between two glass rods instead of as a membrane in a chamber. In all cases, luminal alkalinization is measured by pH stat titration with acid.

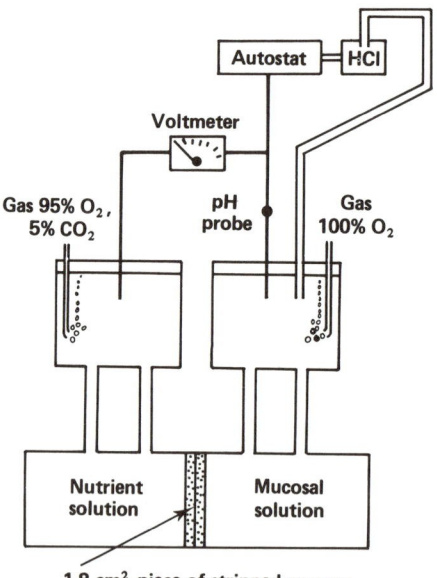

1.8 cm^2 piece of stripped mucosa
suspended as a sheet

Figure 2. Diagrammatic representation of a modified Ussing chamber used for *in vitro* measurement of gastric bicarbonate secretion.

2.2.2. In Vivo

Because antral mucosa does not secrete acid, bicarbonate secretion from surgically created antral pouches can be measured directly. Various methods have been used to inhibit H^+ secretion, permitting measurement of fundic alkali secretion. More recently, methods of simultaneous measurement of gastric HCO_3^- and H^+ secretion have been developed based on the pH and P_{CO_2} of luminal samples. Many species have been studied, including humans (*vide infra*) conscious dogs, cats, rats, and anesthetized guinea pigs. In addition, duodenal bicarbonate secretion has been studied in animals by perfusing an isolated loop of duodenum, with an intact blood supply.

2.2.3. Human Studies

Since 1981, it has been possible to measure gastric bicarbonate secretion in human subjects. Several methods have been used, all relying on the basic reaction

$$H^+ + HCO_3^- = CO_2 + H_2O$$

Perfusion of the stomach with a nonabsorbable marker permits the calculation of gastric volume. Bicarbonate concentration can be calculated from the pH and P_{CO_2} value of the aspirates using the Henderson–Hassalbach equation. A potential problem is gastric contamination with duodenal contents, including bicarbonate-rich pancreatobiliary secretion. Investigators have used different techniques to resolve this, some occluding the pylorus with balloons and others correcting for duodenogastric reflux by simultaneous perfusion of the duodenum with a second marker (Fig. 3). These techniques give quite similar values for gastric bicarbonate secretion: ~450 μmoles/hr. However, more recently a method has been used based on the osmolality change in gastric juice produced by the reaction between H^+ and HCO_3^-. This method does not involve the suppression of acid secretion and gives much higher values for bicarbonate secretion (~2500 μmoles/hr).

Measurement of duodenal bicarbonate secretion is much more difficult and to date has been successfully performed only by Isenberg in the United States. A segment of duodenum is isolated between two balloons, perfused, and the bicarbonate output calculated from the aspirates. This method has shown basal duodenal bicarbonate secretion to be ~150 μmoles/cm per hr.

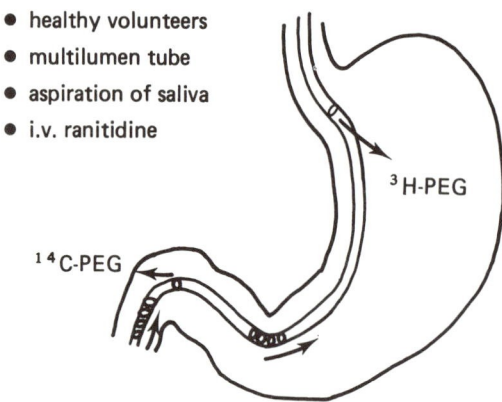

- healthy volunteers
- multilumen tube
- aspiration of saliva
- i.v. ranitidine

^{3}H-PEG

^{14}C-PEG

- samples for marker concentration
- pH & pCO_2 to calculate $[HCO_3^-]$

Figure 3. Method for measuring human gastric bicarbonate secretion. (After Rees *et al.*, 1982.)

2.3. Significance of Bicarbonate Secretion

The existence of alkali secretion by the stomach and proximal duodenum has now been established but, since its magnitude is so small compared with acid output, its physiological significance remains in doubt. If secreted directly into the lumen, the bicarbonate would be overwhelmed by intraluminal acid and would confer little protection to underlying epithelial cells. An unstirred layer that confines the acid–bicarbonate interaction close to the cell surface is therefore essential; evidence has recently emerged that gastric mucus provides such a zone. Although Hollander (1954) and Heatley (1959) had postulated the existence of a mucus gel layer displaying the acid–bicarbonate interaction, proof of its existence was not forthcoming until the past 5 years. The elaborate studies conducted by Allen provided better understanding of mucus structure and function, and in particular helped explain the viscoelastic properties of the gel. Subsequent studies clarified the structure of the gel and its interaction with small ions, such as hydrogen and sodium. Until recently, there were no methods for measuring the mucus gel thickness in unfixed preparations. Two methods have not been published that permit accurate quantitation of the unstirred layer covering the surface epithelium. The first of these approaches used a slit lamp and pachymeter, which is normally used to measure corneal thickness, while the second employed phase-contrast microscopy. Since the first method may also measure fluid covering the gel, recordings of gel thickness by this technique have been greater in magnitude than those by phase-contrast microscopy, which detects the gel layer only. Despite these discrepancies, the methods have clearly documented the existence of a substantial layer of gel, some 5–10 times the height of epithelial cells, which covers the surface of the gastroduodenal mucosa. The thickness of the gel varies greatly (5–200 μm), even in the same specimen, and recent electron microscopic studies have suggested that small defects may normally occur in the layer. It is difficult to reconcile such defects with the physical properties of a liquid gel, which would tend to flow and fill any holes that developed. The mucus gel layer is a dynamic structure and is reduced by mucolytic agents and increased by prostaglandins, stretching of the mucosa and the ulcer-healing drug, carbenoxolone. Experiments on the intraction between mucus gel and small ions have shown that it does not simply act as an unstirred layer of water. The glycoprotein molecules appear to retard the movement of H^+, so that diffusion of such ions across mucus gel is four times slower than through a similar layer of water.

Mucus gel therefore provides an ideal zone for an acid–bicarbonate interaction close to the cell surface. Mucus gel and bicarbonate secretion clearly complement each other in that either alone would confer little mucosal protection. In combination, however, these components prevent direct exposure of the epithelial cells to luminal acid; this has been confirmed experimentally using pH-sensitive microelectrodes advanced across mucus of gastric and duodenal mucosa. Such experiments have shown a marked pH gradient from lumen to cell surface in both the stomach and proximal duodenum of a variety of animals models both *in vivo* (Fig. 4). More recently, the existence of a pH gradient

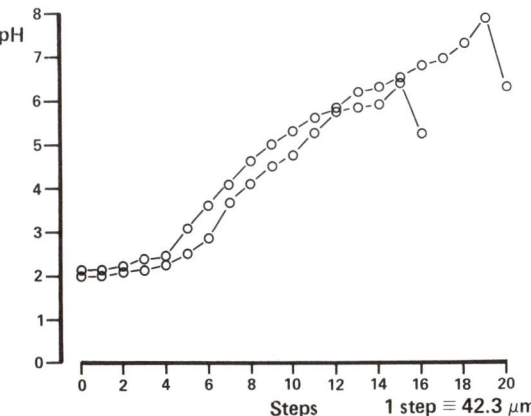

Figure 4. Example of the pH gradient across mucus gel produced by advancing a fine antimony microelectrode from lumen to mucosa. (From Ross *et al.*, 1981.)

between mucosa and gastric lumen has been demonstrated in humans *in vitro* and *in vivo*. In these studies, a fine pH microelectrode was passed down the biopsy channel of an endoscope and advanced from the lumen to rest on mucosa, revealing near neutral juxtamucosal pH despite luminal acidity (Fig. 5). The resulting protective zone produced by bicarbonate transport into mucus gel has been termed the mucus–bicarbonate barrier.

2.4. Mechanisms of Bicarbonate Secretion

How is bicarbonate secreted into the mucus gel layer in order to set up this pH gradient? The mechanisms of secretion are different for stomach and duodenum.

2.4.1. Gastric Bicarbonate Secretion

Bicarbonate is secreted by surface epithelial cells of the stomach at a basal rate of about 5–10% of maximum acid output. Initial experimental work with isolated amphibian mucosa, and more recently with isolated and *in vivo* mammalian preparations, has shown that bicarbonate ions are transported across gastric mucosa by either a metabolically dependent transcellular route or by passive

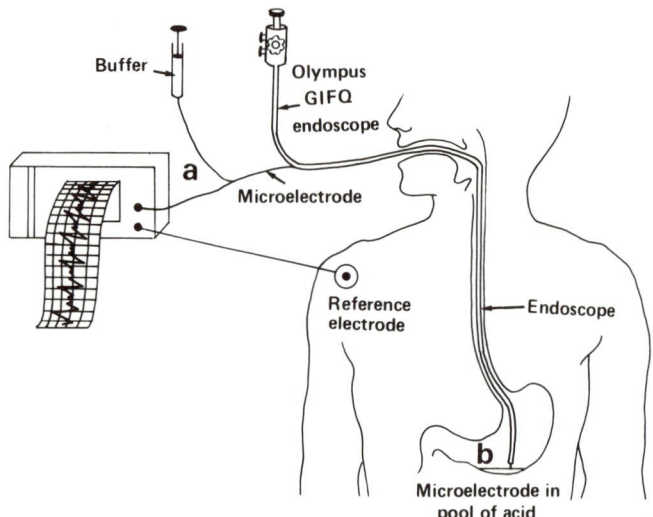

Figure 5. Method used for demonstrating pH gradient between lumen and gastric mucosa in man *in vivo*. (From Quigley and Turnberg, 1987.)

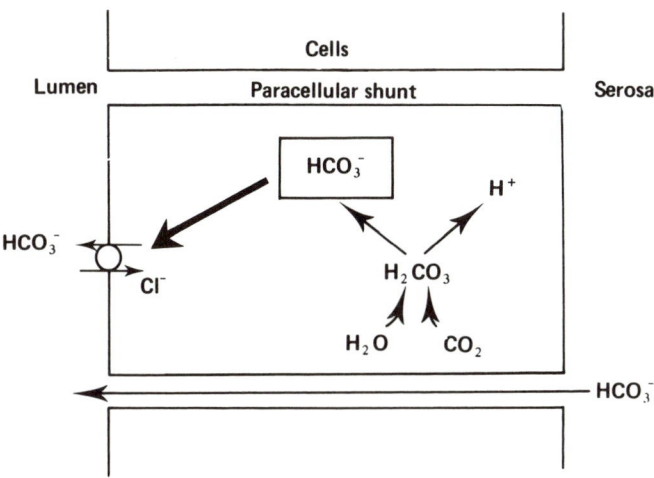

Figure 6. Transport mechanisms for bicarbonate across gastric epithelium.

diffusion through paracellular channels (Fig. 6). The gastric fundus appears to transport bicarbonate by a metabolically dependent process only, secretion being abolished or substantially decreased by anoxia or inhibitors of tissue metabolism (potassium cyanide and dinitrophenol). By contrast, the antrum transports about one third its bicarbonate by passive diffusion. Cellular transport of bicarbonate may occur by an electrogenic process, whereby the transfer of ions across a membrane results in alteration of the potential difference and short circuit current, or by an electroneutral process whereby an ion is exchanged for one of similar charge without altering mucosal potential difference. *In vitro* studies suggest that active bicarbonate secretion by fundus and antrum probably occurs by chloride–bicarbonate exchange at the apical membrane of surface epithelial cells. Thus, the cellular transport of bicarbonate by gastric mucosa may be inhibited by agents that interfere with this ion-exchange process, such as 4-acetamido-4′-isothiocyanatostilbene-2,2′-disulfonic acid (SITS), 4,4′ diisothiocyanatostilbene-2,2′-disulfonic acid (DIDS), and furosemide, or by depleting luminal chloride ions. The bicarbonate necessary for this exchange is probably generated within the fundic cells by the action of carbonic anhydrase, since it has been observed that bicarbonate secretion by intact mucosa and monolayers of surface epithelial cells is more sensitive to luminal than to serosal side administration of acetazolamide, an inhibitor of carbonic anhydrase. In the antrum, however, there is also some evidence that extracellular bicarbonate may be an important source of transported bicarbonate.

2.4.2. Duodenal Bicarbonate Secretion

In the duodenum, the situation appears more complex. It is possible that Brunner's glands contribute to the secretion of epithelial bicarbonate, although some of the characteristics originally attributed to Brunner's gland alkaline secretion, such as inhibition by aspirin or stimulation by vasoactive intestinal polypeptide (VIP) have been demonstrated for duodenal mucosa devoid of these glands. Pancreatobiliary secretion also contributes to net luminal alkali. Isolated duodenal mucosa secretes alkali at about twice the rate of gastric mucosa. As in the gastric antrum, approximately 30–40% of basal secretion is the result of passive diffusion across a transepithelial concentration gradient, while most of the remaining basal secretion occurs by an electrogenic transport process, unlike the chloride–bicarbonate exchange of gastric fundus and antrum (Fig. 7). In the duodenum, endogenous production of bicarbonate by the surface cells contributes little to overall alkalinization, in that acetazolamide in a dose resulting in 99% inhibition of carbonic anhydrase fails to inhibit basal duodenal bicarbonate secretion. In this tissue, extracellular bicarbonate appears to be the primary source of transported alkali. Although basal bicarbonate secretion from proximal duodenal mucosa occurs by these two transport processes, there is evidence that a chloride–bicarbonate exchange mechanism may be activated by certain stimulants, such as the hormones gastric inhibitory polypeptide (GIP), and glucagon, as well as by endogenous opiates.

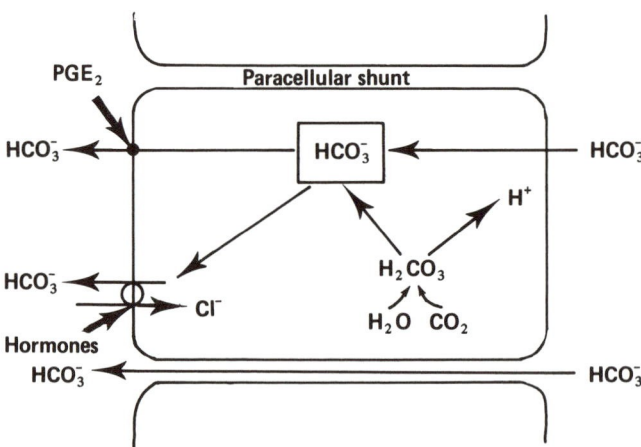

Figure 7. Transport mechanisms for bicarbonate secretion across duodenal epithelium.

3. REGULATION OF GASTRODUODENAL BICARBONATE SECRETION

The demonstration of an alkaline environment adjacent to surface epithelium in the stomach and duodenum and its dependence on mucosal bicarbonate secretion have led to considerable interest in the mechanisms regulating this secretion. A vast amount of information is available on the neurohumoral regulation of gastric acid secretion, but there are comparatively few data on the factors modulating alkali secretion. Furthermore, most of this information has been derived from *in vitro* or *in vivo* studies in which unphysiological amounts of neurotransmitters or hormones have been used to produce a secretory response. Studies on intact animals and the use of physiological stimuli are extremely limited, and it is difficult to decide which of the neurohumoral agents studied play a role in regulating gastroduodenal bicarbonate secretion.

However, recent studies suggest that vagal stimulation and luminal acid probably play an important role in controlling both gastric and duodenal bicarbonate secretion. Gastric bicarbonate secretion may be stimulated by the cholinergic agonist carbachol, and there is evidence that intracellular generation of cyclic guanosine monophosphate (cGMP) and extracellular calcium may also be important. Sham feeding has been shown to increase gastric bicarbonate secretion, while electrical stimulation of the vagi enhances both gastric and duodenal alkalinization. These responses were inhibited by cholinergic antagonists, such as atropine and benzilonium bromide. Further evidence for the neural control of gastroduodenal bicarbonate secretion has been derived from studies in which either electrical stimulation of the nucleus ambiguus or intrahypothalamic infusion of corticotropin-releasing factor have been shown to increase bicarbonate production by stomach or proximal duodenum significantly. Our own studies also suggest an important role for cholinergic neurons in regulating duodenal bicarbonate secretion. Using the technique of electrical field stimulation, we have shown that activation of neurons in isolated duodenal mucosa significantly increases the rate of alkali secretion, a response prevented by atropine. These preliminary observations indicate that vagal cholinergic pathways not only affect gastric acid output but enhance gastroduodenal bicarbonate production as well.

This raises the intriguing possibility that changes in acid output may be coupled with simultaneous changes in gastroduodenal alkali production (Fig. 8). In addition to simultaneous neural stimulation of acid and alkali secretion, there is evidence that other mucosal mechanisms may couple these secretory processes. Using a Heidenhain pouch model, Garner and Hurst (1981) showed that acidification of the gastric remnant resulted in stimulation of bicarbonate secre-

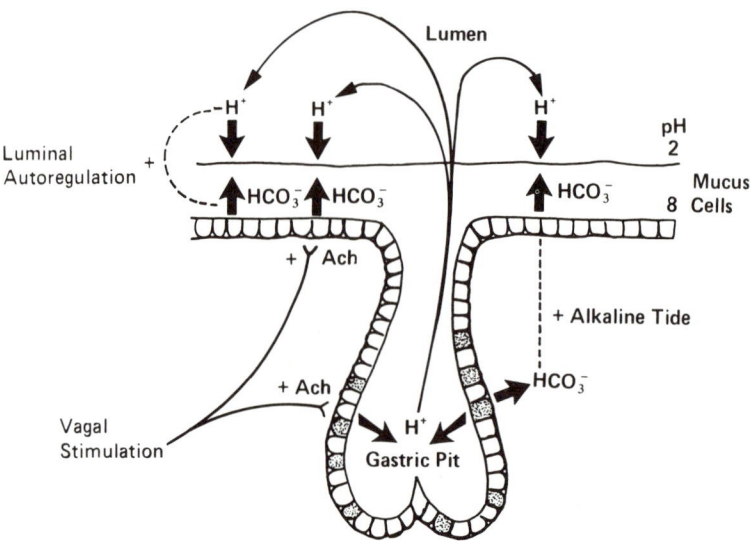

Figure 8. Relationship between acid and alkali secretion.

tion by the pouch. Since the pouch was largely denervated, their results suggest that acidification of gastric mucosa releases a humoral factor that increases bicarbonate production by the surface epithelium, a phenomenon termed autoregulation. In subsequent laboratory studies, Heylings *et al.* confirmed this *in vitro,* using two mucosal strips mounted in parallel in a modified Ussing chamber. In these experiments, there was clearly no neural connection between the mucosa, confirming the release of a factor(s) from one mucosa that acted on the second. Since the response could be reduced by adding indomethacin to the bathing solutions, it was suggested that prostaglandins generated by gastric mucosa exposed to acid were responsible for the alkaline response. The autoregulation of bicarbonate secretion by topical acid has since been demonstrated in both the human stomach and proximal duodenum *in vivo.* Although it has been suggested that the liberation of mucosal prostaglandins may also be responsible for these observations, the evidence is as yet unconvincing. It is possible that in the intact organ, neural mechanisms or other local factors play an important role.

A further link between acid and alkali secretion by gastric mucosa also exists. It has been observed that acid-secreting gastric mucosa is more resistant to damage than is nonsecreting mucosa. Thus, the exposure of gastric mucosa to histamine stimulates acid production and also increases the resistance of the mucosa to damage by intraluminal acid. This response is blocked by H_2-antagonists; it has been suggested that the resistance to damage is produced by the alkaline tide liberated by secreting parietal cells. Release of bicarbonate from parietal cells would in theory provide more interstitial bicarbonate for transport by the surface epithelium. Studies of gastric microvascular casts have demonstrated the existence of capillary loops that would transport bicarbonate liberated by the parietal cells to surface epithelial cells. Furthermore, parenteral infusion of bicarbonate has been shown to protect gastric mucosa from damage. The possibility thus exists that the secretory activity of parietal cells is coupled with the secretory activity of surface epithelial cells via changes in interstitial bicarbonate delivery. Clearly, further studies are necessary to substantiate this theory.

The importance of other neurohumoral factors in regulating gastroduodenal bicarbonate secretion remains uncertain. The gastrointestinal (GI) hormones cholecystokinin (CCK), pancreatic glucagon, and GIP influence gastric alkalinization, while in the duodenum VIP and GIP, but not secretin, have been shown to stimulate output. Norepinephrine and isoproterenol also modify gastroduodenal alkali secretion, and these responses have been incriminated in the pathogenesis of stress ulceration. However, as yet, the physiological or pathological significance of these preliminary experimental observations remains uncertain. The stomach and duodenum have been shown to contain enkephalin-like immunoreactivity in both mucosal endocrine cells and neurons. Recently, two groups of investigators have shown stimulation of duodenal bicarbonate secretion by opioids, and the possibility exists that endogenous opiates also regulate duodenal alkalinization.

It is obvious from the above discussion that the control of gastroduodenal bicarbonate secretion is poorly understood. It seems inevitable that investigators will need to follow the painstaking trail of physiologists and clinicians who helped clarify the regulatory mechanisms for acid secretion.

4. EFFECTS OF DAMAGING AND PROTECTIVE AGENTS ON THE ALKALINE MICROCLIMATE

4.1. Damaging Agents

Although bicarbonate secretion increases with increasing luminal acidity, providing an autoregulatory mechanism boosting the mucus–bicarbonate barrier, at pH <1.5, this protective barrier fails to maintain near-neutral juxtamucosal pH. It is therefore possible that agents cause gastroduodenal damage by adverse effects on bicarbonate secretion. NSAID owe their anti-inflammatory properties to an ability to inhibit synthesis of prostaglandins, which are important mediators of the inflammatory response. Depletion of endogenous prostaglandins would be expected to impair many aspects of mucosal defense. NSAID have been shown to reduce both gastric and duodenal bicarbonate secretion in many animal models, and more recently in humans (Fig. 9). In addition, they have been shown to reduce the pH gradient across gastroduodenal mucosa. Such effects can be prevented by pretreatment with prostaglandins. NSAID, however, influence many components of mucosal defense; reduction in bicarbonate secretion is just one possible mechanism whereby these agents produce damage.

Bile salts, particularly sodium taurocholate, are also potent inhibitors of gastric bicarbonate secretion and have been shown to reduce the pH gradient across mucus gel. As in NSAID, this effect may be important in producing mucosal damage. Ethanol also inhibits gastric bicarbonate secretion although this is unlikely to be an important mechanism of damage as ethanol passes easily through the mucus–bicarbonate barrier to the underlying mucosa.

4.2. Protective Agents

Exogenous prostaglandins have been shown to protect gastric mucosa from the effects of a variety of damaging agents. Local generation of these substances within gastric mucosa has also been considered responsible for mucosal adaptation to attack by mild irritants (adaptive cytoprotection), although some current evidence suggests that adaptive cytoprotection may occur independent of prostaglandins. It has been shown that prostaglandins enhance the mucus–bicarbonate barrier; there is evidence that both the mucus gel and bicarbonate secretion

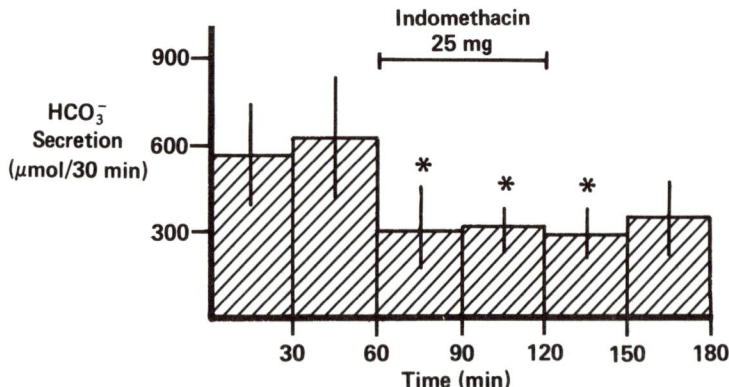

Figure 9. Effect of indomethacin 25 mg on bicarbonate output by the healthy human stomach.

components are influenced by these agents. More detailed analysis of the information, however, demonstrates a number of important flaws in the hypothesis. First, a number of prostaglandins protect gastroduodenal mucosa without influencing bicarbonate secretion. Second, careful microscopic evaluation of the protective effect of exogenous prostaglandins against damage by various topical agents suggests that the surface epithelium is not protected and that the major impact of such prostaglandins is submucosal. This would suggest that, under such circumstances, prostaglandin-mediated effects on the mucus–bicarbonate barrier contribute little to overall mucosal protection. This is particularly relevant for ethanol induced mucosal damage. Finally, although certain ulcer-healing drugs may produce simultaneous increases in prostaglandin formation and bicarbonate secretion by gastroduodenal mucosa, there is conflicting evidence that these two processes are causally linked.

There is no doubt that certain exogenous prostaglandins increase both mucus gel thickness and bicarbonate secretion, leading to an enhanced pH gradient overlying gastric and duodenal epithelium. The importance of endogenous prostaglandin metabolism in the physiological control of bicarbonate secretion remains uncertain, and as yet there is insufficient evidence to link prostaglandin-induced mucosal protection to enhancement of the mucus–bicarbonate barrier. It has been established that prostaglandins influence a number of other protective mechanisms, such as surface-active phospholipids and mucosal blood flow, and these different protective mechanisms may be called into action to deal with different damaging agents or even different concentrations of the same agent. Thus, prostaglandin-induced enhancement of the mucus–bicarbonate barrier may be important in protecting against acid and NSAID (depending on local concentrations) but is of little significance in preventing damage by ethanol.

5. IMPORTANCE OF THE ALKALINE MICROCLIMATE IN THE PATHOGENESIS AND TREATMENT OF PEPTIC ULCER DISEASE

Although there is evidence that mucosal damage by bile salts and NSAID may, in part, be mediated by the adverse effects of these agents on the mucus–bicarbonate barrier, there is very little information to link defects in the barrier with peptic ulcer pathogenesis (Fig. 10).

The mucus gel structure in gastric ulcer patients has been demonstrated to be abnormal in that it contains less native glycoprotein, while certain pepsins, which are more prevalent in duodenal ulcer disease, are capable of more ag-

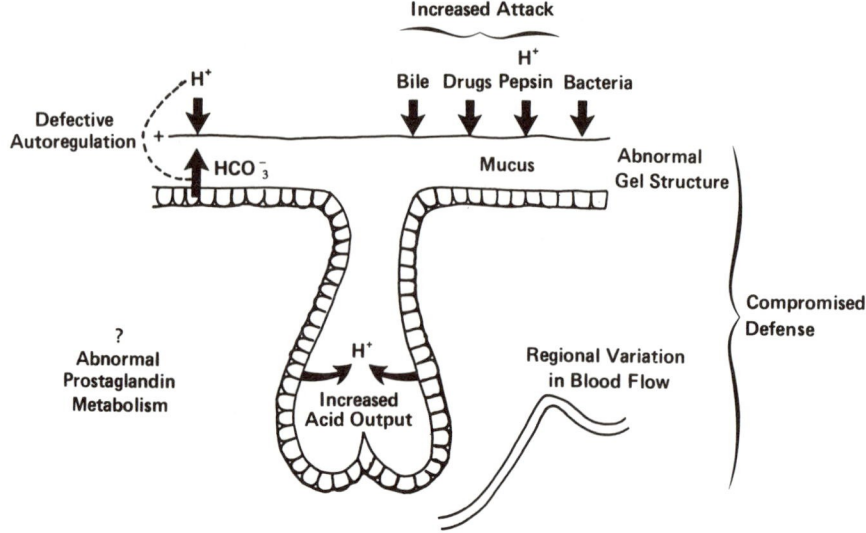

Figure 10. Possible role of mucosal defense mechanisms in the pathogenesis of peptic ulcer disease.

gressive digestion of the glycoprotein matrix. In duodenal ulcer, the bicarbonate response to an acid load is defective and an abnormal pH gradient in response to luminal acid has also been demonstrated in these patients. This indicates a defect in the ability of these patients to maintain juxtamucosal neutrality in the face of luminal acidity. Although this evidence points to a link between abnormalities of the mucus–bicarbonate barrier and ulcer pathogenesis, this generalized defect in the barrier cannot explain the focal nature of chronic peptic ulcer disease and its predisposition for certain anatomical sites. Similarly, this argument applies to other protective zones, such as surface-active phospholipids (gastric only), impermeability of the apical cell membrane–intercellular junctions, and restitution. However, coupled with regional variations in blood flow, which would predispose certain areas to damage by acid, such generalized abnormalities may result in focal injury.

Once such an ulcer has formed, the normal mucus–bicarbonate barrier disappears from ulcerated tissue and is replaced with a layer of sloughed epithelial cells, fibrin and mucus covering the damaged mucosa, into which diffuses alkali from interstitial tissue. The healing of such chronic ulcers is poorly understood but is likely to be a complex process that is dependent on the re-establishment of the mucosal vasculature and connective tissue matrix, followed by re-epithelialization. A number of drugs have been shown to accelerate the rate of this healing process; the mode of action of those that do not inhibit acid secretion remains uncertain.

In some instances, the ulcer-healing action has been linked to effects on gastroduodenal bicarbonate secretion. Prostaglandin analogues have recently been introduced as antiulcer drugs and have been shown to stimulate gastric and duodenal alkalinization under certain experimental conditions. It is conceivable that their therapeutic action depends, in part, on this enhancement of the mucus–bicarbonate barrier. There is also evidence that some of the other currently available antiulcer drugs influence the mucus–bicarbonate barrier. The antacid aluminum has been shown to produce marked stimulation of gastroduodenal alkali secretion in isolated mucosae. This observation is quite intriguing, as it implies that in addition to providing an exogenous source of alkali to neutralize luminal acid, aluminum-containing antacids may also enhance the delivery of endogenous alkali into the mucus gel layer. Sucralfate and colloidal bismuth have also been shown to have similar effects in isolated mucosae, and more recently in humans. Since sucralfate contains aluminum, it is tempting to speculate that a common denominator to these agents is a metallic cation. How these agents enhance alkali secretion remains uncertain, however, and there is conflicting information on the involvement of endogenous prostaglandin metabolism.

Although prostaglandins and these other ulcer-healing agents enhance the normal mucus–bicarbonate barrier overlying healthy epithelium, it is difficult to envisage the importance this would have in accelerating chronic ulcer healing. It seems more realistic to propose that enhancement of the mucus–bicarbonate barrier would be of greater value in ulcer prophylaxis. A strengthened barrier would theoretically prevent recurrence of peptic ulcer after initial healing, prevent NSAID-induced damage, or stress ulceration in severely ill patients. This principle may also apply to other defense mechanisms, such as surface hydrophobicity, the epithelial cell barrier to ionic diffusion, and epithelial cell migration. There is little doubt that the prophylactic effect of exogenous prostaglandins is largely dependent on maintaining microvascular integrity.

ACKNOWLEDGMENTS. The authors are grateful to the Department of Medical Illustration, Hope Hospital, for providing the figures. Dr. Shorrock is a British Society of Gastroenterology Research Fellow.

ANNOTATED BIBLIOGRAPHY

Bickel M, Kaufman G: Gastric mucus gel thickness: Effect of distension, 16,16-dimethylprostaglandin E2 and carbenoxolone. *Gastroenterology* **80:**770–775, 1981.
Method for measuring mucus gel thickness and the effects of various agents on this thickness.

Flemstrom G: Gastric and duodenal mucosal bicarbonate secretion, in Johnson RL, Christensen J, Jacobson E, Jackson MJ, Walsh JH (eds): *Physiology of the GI tract,* ed. 2. Vol. 2. New York, Raven, 1986. pp. 1011–1029.

Thorough discussion of physiology and measurement of mucosal bicarbonate secretion.

Flemstrom G, Kivilaakso E: Demonstration of a pH gradient at the luminal surface of rat duodenum in vivo and its dependence on mucosal alkaline secretion. *Gastroenterology* **84:**787–794, 1983.

Important paper demonstrating duodenal pH gradient in vivo.

Heatley NG: Mucosubstance and a barrier to diffusion. *Gastroenterology* **37:**313–317, 1959.

Classic paper predicting the presence of the mucus–bicarbonate barrier.

Heylings JR, Garner A, Flemstrom G: Regulation of gastroduodenal bicarbonate transport by luminal acid in the frog in vitro. *Am J Physiol* **246:**G235–242, 1984.

Important paper introducing the concept of autoregulation of bicarbonate secretion.

Isenberg JI, Hogan DL, Koss MA, et al: Human duodenal mucosal bicarbonate secretion. Evidence for basal secretion and stimulation by hydrochloric acid and a synthetic prostaglandin E1 analogue. *Gastroenterology* **91:**370–378, 1986.

Shows method for measuring human duodenal bicarbonate secretion.

Quigley EMM, Turnberg LA: The pH of the microclimate lining human gastric and duodenal mucosa in vivo: Studies in control subjects and in duodenal ulcer patients. *Gastroenterology* **92:**1876–1884, 1987.

Shows method used for measuring pH gradient in human gastric and duodenal mucosa.

Rees WDW, Botham D, Turnberg LA: A demonstration of bicarbonate production by the normal human stomach in vivo. *Dig Dis Sci* **27:**961–966, 1982.

Important paper showing method for measuring human gastric bicarbonate secretion.

Rees WDW, Gibbons LC, Warhurst G, et al: Studies of bicarbonate secretion in the normal human stomach in vivo: Effect of aspirin, sodium taurocholate, and prostaglandin E2, in Allen A, Flemstrom G, Garner A, Silen W, Turnberg, LA (eds): *Mechanisms of Mucosal Protection in the Upper Gastrointestinal Tract.* New York, Raven, 1984, p. 119–123.

Shows effect of various damaging and protective agents on human gastric bicarbonate secretion.

Ross IN, Bahari HMM, Turnberg LA: The pH gradient across mucus adherent to rat fundic mucosa in vivo and the effects of possible damaging agents. *Gastroenterology* **81:**713–718, 1981.

Important paper showing measurement of pH gradient across gastric mucus gel and the effect of damaging agents.

Schierbeck NP: Ueber Kohlemsaure im Ventrikel. *Scand Arch Physiol* **8:**437–474, 1892.

Classic work of historical interest.

Wallace JL, Whittle BJR: Role of mucus in the repair of gastric epithelial damage in the rat. *Gastroenterology* **91:**603–611, 1986.

Important paper discussing the importance of the mucus cap.

7

Epithelial Cell Renewal

GREGORY L. EASTWOOD

1. INTRODUCTION

The epithelium of the gastrointestinal (GI) tract undergoes constant rapid renewal. This process is an important mechanism of mucosal protection throughout the GI tract because it maintains the functional integrity of the epithelium and is also necessary for the repair of mucosal injury. Thus, it is reasonable to expect that certain conditions and agents that predispose to peptic ulcer disease or mucosal injury may do so in part by affecting epithelial renewal in the upper GI tract.

A century ago, the Italian anatomist Bizzozero predicted the phenomenon of epithelial renewal on the basis of mitotic counts in light microscopic histologic sections of small intestinal mucosa. However, an appreciation of the details of epithelial cell kinetics had to await the application of autoradiographic methods in the 1950s. Since then, we have learned a great deal about the process of normal epithelial renewal, its regulation, and its alteration by physiological events, disease states, and so-called ulcerogenic agents.

GREGORY L. EASTWOOD • Gastroenterology Division, University of Massachusetts Medical School, Worcester, Massachusetts 01605.

2. EPITHELIAL RENEWAL IN THE NORMAL GASTROINTESTINAL TRACT

2.1. Process of Epithelial Renewal

The total process of epithelial renewal involves the proliferation, migration, differentiation, senescence, and eventual loss of GI epithelial cells. Proliferation occurs within more or less discrete zones throughout the GI tract (Fig. 1). Within these proliferative zones, undifferentiated cells divide to provide a constant source of new cells, which, with some exceptions, then migrate toward the gut lumen, into which they eventually are extruded. The lowermost four to five cells within the proliferative zone of the small intestine, including the duodenum, are called stem cells. Presumably, stem cells also are located within the proliferative zones of the stomach and esophagus, but they have not yet been identified. In the small intestine, cells within the stem cell area divide, migrate up within the proliferative zone, and then divide further. When cells migrate beyond the proliferative zone, they lose the ability to divide and become differentiated to carry out the specialized functions of that portion of the GI tract wherein they arise.

During the process of cell division, cells undergo a sequence of phases known as the cell renewal cycle (Fig. 2). Upon completion of mitosis (M phase),

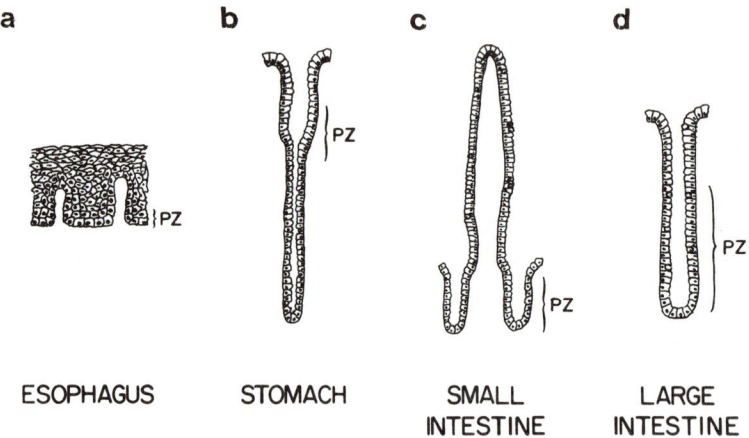

Figure 1. Proliferative zone (PZ) in each major region of the gastrointestinal tract. (a) Esophagus, PZ is confined to the basal cell layer. (b) Stomach, PZ is located at the top of the glands and the base of the pits. (c) Small intestine. (d) Large intestine. PZ is in the lower portions of the crypts. (From Eastwood, 1977.)

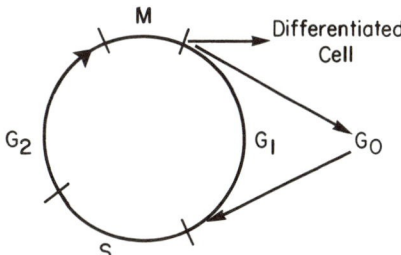

Figure 2. Cell renewal cycle. G_1, postmitotic–presynthetic gap; S, DNA synthesis; G_2, post-synthetic–premitotic gap; M, mitosis; G_0, prolonged G_1. (From Eastwood, 1977.)

proliferating cells enter the first portion of interphase called the postmitotic–presynthetic gap, or G_1 phase. DNA replication ensues during the DNA synthesis (S) phase. This is followed by another interval, the postsynthetic–premitotic gap, or G_2 phase, before mitosis occurs again. After mitosis, some cells may enter a prolonged G_1 phase, called the G_0 phase, during which DNA synthesis and mitosis are temporarily suspended, but the potential for cell division remains. Other cells, on completion of mitosis, migrate out of the proliferative zone, relinquish the ability to proliferate, and differentiate into mature epithelial cells.

The duration of each of the phases within the cell cycle has been estimated using autoradiographic methods. Durations vary from one region of the GI tract to another but, in general, M phase requires about 1 hr, G_1 phase about 10–15 hr, S phase about 10 hr, and G_2 phase 1–6 hr. The total duration of the cell cycle in human GI epithelium is about 1–2 days.

The events of the cell cycle are accompanied by great metabolic activity. Although DNA synthesis occurs only during a discrete period, synthesis of RNA and protein is active throughout the cell cycle, except during M phase. During G_1 phase, the replication of new DNA is anticipated by the synthesis of enzymes involved in nucleic acid metabolism, such as thymidine kinase.

2.2. Epithelial Renewal within the Esophagus, Stomach, and Duodenum

2.2.1. Esophagus

The epithelium of the esophagus differs from the epithelia found elsewhere within the GI tract. In the esophagus, the epithelium is stratified squamous, whereas between the esophagogastric junction and the anus, the tubular lumen is lined by columnar epithelium, which is only one cell thick, but convoluted into ridges, villi, glands, and the other architectural characteristics of the stomach and intestine. In the stratified squamous epithelium of the esophagus, papillae of the lamina propria project into the esophageal epithelium at irregular intervals similar to the rete pegs that project into the stratified squamous epithelium of the skin. Small esophageal mucus-secreting glands, composed of cuboidal and columnar cells, are located beneath the epithelium in the upper esophagus and near the esophagogastric junction.

The stratified squamous epithelium of the esophagus is subdivided into three layers: the superficial stratum corneum, the intermediate stratum spinosum, and the basal stratum germinativum. The proliferative zone in the esophagus is the stratum germinativum, a layer of polygonal cells that is applied to the basement membrane overlying the lamina propria (see Fig. 1). Autoradiographic studies indicate that cells leave the basal layer in a random fashion and migrate toward the lumen. In rodents, replacement of the esophageal epithelium takes about 7 days. In humans, renewal of the epithelium probably requires about 2 weeks.

2.2.2. Stomach

The mucosa of the stomach is divided into two types that differ in structure and function. Fundic type mucosa lines the body and fundus and antral type lines the antrum. In fundic type mucosa, mucus-secreting cells are found on the surface, extending down into the gastric pits. Beneath the pits and emptying into them are long convoluted glands lined by parietal cells, which secrete acid and intrinsic factor, and chief cells, which secrete pepsinogens. In antral mucosa, mucus-secreting cells also line the surface and the elongated pits, but the glandular cells beneath the pits elaborate an alkaline mucus that contains pepsinogens. Endocrine cells are found in the glands of both antral and fundic type mucosa. In particular, the hormone gastrin is secreted from G cells located in the glands of the antrum.

The proliferative zone of the gastric epithelium is located at the base of the pits and the contiguous upper portion of the glands (see Fig. 1). Cells migrate upward into the pits and onto the mucosal surface to replenish the surface mucous cells. Renewal of this population takes about 2–7 days in humans.

Cells also migrate downward from the proliferative zone to replenish the parietal and chief cells within the gastric glands. Renewal of the glandular epithelium of the stomach is much slower than that of the surface epithelium, probably requiring several months. The fate of senescent glandular cell is not known.

2.2.3. Duodenum

A continuous single-cell-thick layer of epithelium covers the villi and lines the crypts of the duodenum and the rest of the small intestine. In the jejunum, the ratio of villous height to crypt depth is about 5:1. However, in the proximal duodenum, because of distortions related to acid, bile, and other secretions, the villi may appear shorter, broader, and irregular. Four major epithelial cell types have been identified in small intestinal epithelium: absorptive cells, mucus-secreting cells (goblet cells), Paneth cells, and enteroendocrine cells.

Absorptive cells: These cells originate at the base of the crypts as immature proliferative cells, differentiate as they migrate up the crypts onto the villi, and finally are extruded from the villous tips into the bowel lumen. In humans, this renewal process requires about 1 week.

Mucus cells: These cells also originate in the multipotential proliferative cells in the lower crypts and migrate with the absorptive cells to the villous tips.

Paneth cells: These cells are found predominantly at the base of the crypts. They do not appear to migrate but presumably develop from cells in the proliferative zone in the lower portion of the crypts. They contain granules that appear red by hematoxylin and eosin (H & E) staining. They probably have a secretory function, as yet unidentified.

Enteroendocrine cells: These cells also appear to arise from undifferentiated crypt cells and migrate to the villous tips. A wide variety of endocrine cells have been described, including cells that secrete gastrin, cholecystokinin (CCK), secretin, somatostatin, and gastric inhibitory polypeptide.

2.3. Regulation of Epithelial Renewal

The regulation of GI epithelial renewal is a complex process that involves the interaction of numerous extracellular factors with the intracellular control mechanisms for proliferation, migration, differentiation, and cell loss. The presence of food in the gut stimulates epithelial proliferation. During starvation, the synthesis of DNA, the proliferation and migration of epithelial cells, and the thickness of the mucosa all are decreased. On refeeding, these changes reverse. Are these effects of starvation the result of lack of food in the gut or of general protein-calorie malnutrition? Apparently they are related more to lack of intraluminal food than to starvation per se because studies in intravenously alimented animals also show that epithelial proliferation and migration are depressed and that the mucosa becomes thinner.

The effects of food on epithelial renewal may be hormonally mediated. Intravenous alimentation of rats is associated with profound decreases in antral gastrin concentrations, but infusions of pentagastrin during intravenous alimentation will prevent the expected decreases in both GI tissue weight and disaccharidase activity. Ample evidence from other animal studies indicates that gastrin is trophic for gastric fundic and duodenal mucosae. In humans, gastric mucosal hyperplasia, which primarily involves the parietal cell mass, commonly accompanies the hypergastrinemia of Zollinger–Ellison (Z–E) syndrome.

Other hormones and agents also appear to stimulate epithelial proliferation, including CCK, enteroglucagon, epidermal growth factor (EGF), and bile salts. Thus, although food in the gut may have some direct effect on epithelial renewal, eating produces a variety of effects that influence the process.

Corticosteroids have been shown to inhibit proliferation and to retard migration of epithelial cells. This has been invoked to explain why corticosteroids may predispose to ulcer formation and interfere with ulcer healing. The effects of corticosteroids on epithelial proliferation are discussed further in Section 4.

Prostaglandins are thought to be important in conferring so-called cytoprotective properties on the mucosa of the upper GI tract—but do they have any effect on epithelial renewal? Administration of prostaglandins of the E series results in a thickening of the gastric mucosa. However, the evidence thus far indicates that the cytoprotective prostaglandins probably do not have a primary effect on epithelial proliferation but rather retard cell loss, which leads to an accumulation of epithelial cells and thickening of the mucosa.

The mesenchyme in the lamina propria that underlies the epithelium also appears to play an important role in regulation of epithelial renewal. The crypts of small intestinal mucosa are surrounded by a sheath of fibroblasts that undergo proliferation and migration to the upper portions of the crypts in synchrony with epithelial migration. The fibroblasts continue to migrate to the villous tips, perhaps at an accelerated rate compared with epithelial migration. Both *in vivo* and *in vitro* studies indicate that the subepithelial mesenchyme is necessary for normal epithelial renewal.

Finally, local regulation of epithelial renewal involves the feedback control of proliferation within the proliferative zones by the rate of cell loss on the mucosal surface. When the villous cell population is selectively diminished by experimental ischemia in rats, proliferation is stimulated. Conversely, abundant numbers of villous epithelial cells or retardation of loss of cells from the mucosal surface appear to inhibit epithelial proliferation. Undoubtedly, a similar local regulation of proliferation operates in the stomach and esophagus.

2.4. Restitution of the Epithelium

Restitution refers to the ability of denuded superficial epithelium to reconstitute itself within minutes to hours after the initial injury. This phenomenon has been described most completely in rat gastric mucosa exposed briefly (typically for less than 1 min) to 100% ethanol. After cessation of the ethanol exposure, much of the epithellum in the upper portion of the gastric pits and on the mucosal surface lifts off into the gastric lumen, leaving a bare lamina propria. Within several minutes, however, epithelial cells begin to migrate upward from the deeper portion of the gastric pits by extending long lamellae over the exposed basement membrane. By 30–60 min postinjury, this process has succeeded in covering the mucosal surface again with epithelium.

The phenomenon of restitution is probably responsible for the immediate healing of small areas of superficial damage to the epithelium, damage that may occur as a result of minor trauma from food ingestion or irritating agents. Restitution does not immediately involve the proliferation of new epithelial cells, although it is likely that conditions that would provoke a continued or repeated process of restitution would eventually stimulate proliferation.

3. METHODS OF STUDYING EPITHELIAL RENEWAL

3.1. Light Microscopy

Ordinary light microscopic histologic sections can be used to measure mucosal thickness and other architectural aspects of the mucosa, such as crypt depth and villous height in duodenal mucosa. Mitotic counts, although tedious, can be used to estimate epithelial proliferation but are of no use in studying migration or cell loss.

3.2. Radioactive Labeling of Newly Synthesized DNA with Tritiated Thymidine

When tritiated thymidine, $[^3H]$-TdR, is injected into animals or exposed to biopsies of human GI mucosa, it is rapidly incorporated into newly synthesized DNA and thus can be used to label proliferating cells. Although the physical half-life of tritium is about 12 years, the biological availability of [³H]-TdR is limited to about $\frac{1}{2}$ hr. This makes [³H]-TdR an ideal pulse label for a cohort of proliferating cells. Epithelial renewal using [³H]-TdR can be studied in two ways: autoradiography and scintillation counting of radioactive DNA.

Autoradiography is a photographic technique that offers more specific information about proliferation and migration of epithelial cells but is less sensitive than measurement of radiolabeled DNA. Light microscopic autoradiographs are made by dipping histologic tissue sections that contain [³H]-TdR in photographic emulsion, such that a thin layer of emulsion overlies the section. The β-emissions from the nuclei that have incorporated the [³H]-TdR expose the silver granules above the labeled nucleus and, after development of the emulsion, appear as clusters of black granules over labeled nuclei (Fig. 3). Autoradiographs prepared 1 hr after exposure of the tissue to [³H]-TdR can be used to provide information about proliferation. Autoradiographs prepared one or more days later can provide information about migration of epithelial cells because the radioactive label will remain within the nuclei as the cells migrate to the mucosal surface and are lost into the gut lumen.

For example, to measure proliferation using autoradiographic methods: (1) the size of the proliferative zone can be estimated by the identifying the locations of labeled cells, (2) the fraction of the mucosal thickness or of the crypt depth occupied by the proliferative zone can be documented, and (3) the number of labeled cells can be counted. To study migration, the distance that labeled cells have migrated toward the mucosal surface can be measured.

Extraction of DNA from [³H]-TdR-labeled tissues also can be used to estimate proliferation. Although this method will detect more subtle differences than will autoradiography, it does not provide information about the location of proliferating cells. Furthermore, all cells, both epithelial and mesenchymal, that are synthesizing DNA at the time the [³H]-TdR is available will incorporate the label. Thus, the specific activity of radiolabeled DNA is perhaps a relection of, but not specific for, epithelial proliferation.

3.3. Measurement of Substances Involved in Cell Growth

The polyamines, putrescine, spermidine, and spermine, are distributed throughout living tissue and appear to be important in cellular growth. During cell proliferation, polyamines are synthesized and accumulate in growing tissues. Putrescine is formed from ornithine in a reaction catalyzed by ornithine decarboxylase (ODC); putrescine is further converted to spermidine and then to spermine. Because ODC is the rate limiting enzyme of the polyamine synthetic

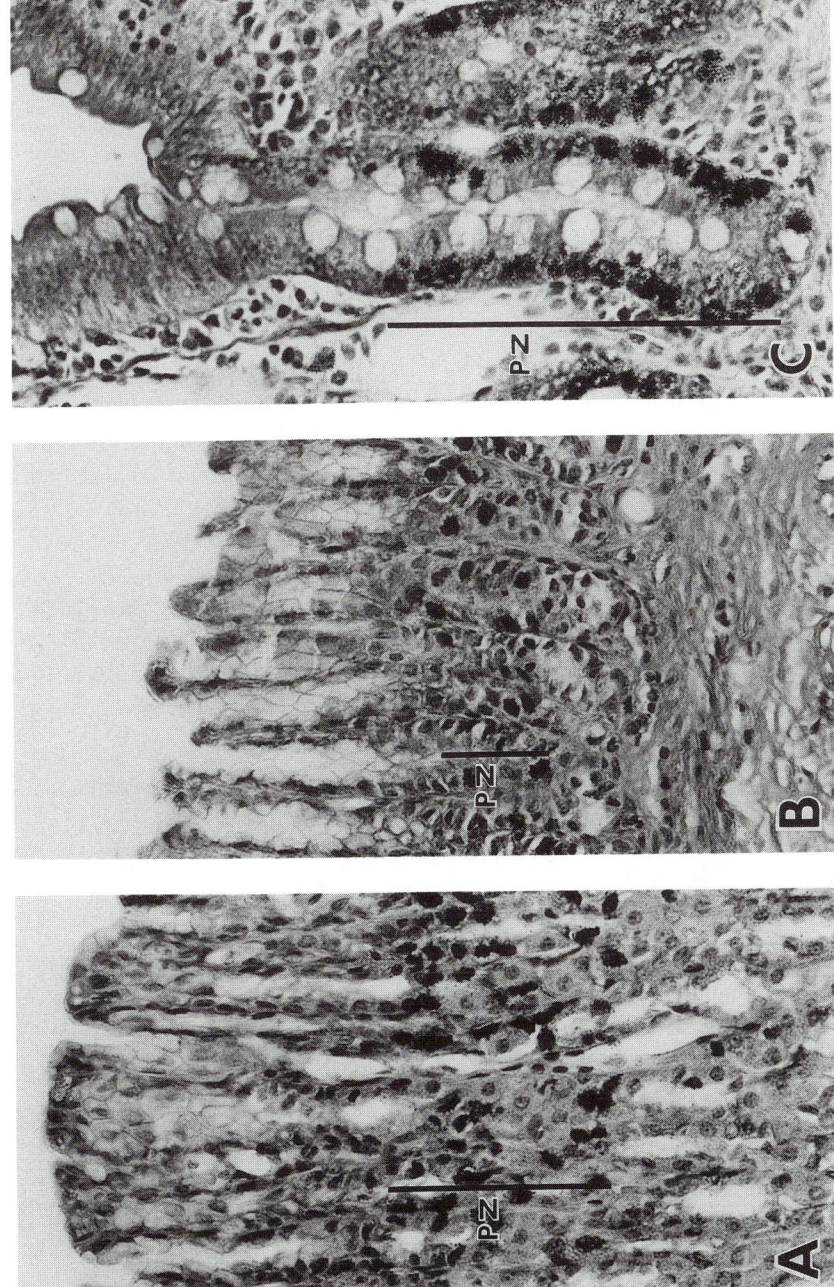

Figure 3. Photomicrographs of autoradiographs from rat fundic (A), antral (B), and duodenal (C) mucosae. The clusters of black granules identify nuclei that have incorporated tritiated thymidine. PZ, proliferative zones (cf. Fig. 1).

pathway and because increased ODC activity correlates well with rapid cell growth, it has been used to study epithelial proliferation in the GI tract. Measurement of enzymes, such as thymidine kinase, that are important in the synthesis of DNA, have also been used to estimate proliferation.

4. EPITHELIAL RENEWAL IN DISORDERS OF THE ESOPHAGUS, STOMACH, AND DUODENUM

4.1. Esophagus

A common histologic finding in esophageal mucosal biopsies from patients with gastroesophageal reflux disease is thickening of the basal layer of epithelial cells. Because the basal layer comprises the zone of proliferating cells, the expanded basal layer is perhaps attributable to stimulation of epithelial proliferation by irritating refluxed material. This has been verified by [3H]-TdR) autoradiographic studies of biopsies from patients with reflux disease, which showed that proliferation was markedly stimulated compared with control subjects. Another study showed that a single instillation of 0.0025 N HCl into the esophagus of dogs for 30 min resulted in an increase in [3H]-TdR-labeled cells 16 hr later and a peak in mitoses at 20 hr. Thus, it appears that the stimulation of epithelial proliferation in reflux disease is a protective response to acid or other refluxed material. Epithelial proliferation in Barrett's epithelium, a columnar metaplasia of the esophagus that develops as a consequence of chronic gastroesophageal reflux, is discussed in Section 5.

4.2. Stomach and Duodenum

Experimental gastric injury apears to stimulate epithelial renewal. When aspirin is administered to rats, superficial areas of injury that do not extend down to the proliferative zone heal rapidly, within 24 hr, perhaps because of the process of restitution (see Section 2.4). By contrast, deeper aspirin lesions that involve the proliferative zone do stimulate proliferation and may take up to 10 days to heal. Similarly, acute alcohol injury in both animals and humans is associated with a stimulation of epithelial proliferation.

A number of studies have looked at the effects of chronic ingestion of ulcerogens on epithelial proliferation. In rats given aspirin in their drinking water for 4 weeks at a concentration that causes no gross or histologic injury, epithelial proliferation is stimulated in the fundic mucosa but not in the antrum. Chronic indomethacin ingestion in rats and humans has similar effects. The stimulatory effect of these agents on fundic epithelial proliferation may be relevant to the observation that the gastric mucosa appears to adapt to repeated administration of aspirin. It is a well-observed phenomenon that chronic administration of aspirin to rats and humans results in a decrease in the susceptibility of the gastric mucosa to the injurious effects of aspirin. Furthermore, aspirin and indomethacin are more likely to cause erosions and ulcerations in the antrum. Thus, it is possible that the failure of antral epithelial proliferation to respond to aspirin or indomethacin may account in part for the ulcerogenic action of these drugs.

Ethanol, in the form of beer, taken as one bottle a night for 2 weeks, appears to stimulate human fundic epithelial proliferation but has no effect in the antrum. These findings are similar to those observed after aspirin and indomethacin. However, in rats that received a chronically low concentration (15%) of ethanol, there was no measurable effect on proliferation in either fundic or antral mucosa. Thus, the effects of chronic ethanol ingestion on epithelial proliferation are inconclusive.

In contrast to the effects of aspirin and indomethacin, and perhaps of ethanol, on epithelial proliferation, corticosteroids have been shown to depress epithelial proliferation in both rats and humans. Steroids do not cause direct injury to the mucosa of the upper GI tract, and their role in the pathogenesis of peptic disease has been debated. Nevertheless, the inhibition of epithelial proliferation by steroids could relate to the pathogenesis of peptic disease in at least two ways. First, the normal process of epithelial renewal would be impaired, rendering the mucosa susceptible to the effects of other ulcerogens. Second, the healing of existing mucosal lesions would be retarded.

In addition to the effects of the potential ulcerogens, aspirin, indomethacin, ethanol, and corticosteroids, the effects of psychophysiologic stress on epithelial proliferation have also been studied. In rats subjected to water-immersion restraint–stress, epithelial proliferation is depressed in the fundic mucosa. Although it is reasonable to expect that circulating levels of corticosteroids will be high during stress, numerous other factors may affect epithelial proliferation and the other mechanisms of mucosal protection. Nevertheless, stress-related gastric erosions are more likely to occur in fundic mucosa. It is interesting to speculate whether there might be a causal relationship between stress-induced depression of epithelial proliferation and the development of fundic lesions in humans, such as may occur in very ill patients in intensive care units.

If epithelial proliferation appears to be stimulated in response to acute gastric mucosal injury and chronic exposure to some acute ulcerogens, what are the characteristics of epithelial proliferation in chronic gastritis? Chronic gastritis is actually a somewhat arbitrary designation for a spectrum of histopathological findings that range from infiltration of the lamina propria with chronic inflammatory cells through mild thinning of the mucosa to frank gastric atrophy, with marked thinning of the mucosa, attenuation of the glands, and loss of parietal and chief cells. Despite the apparent atrophy, it is of interest that the activity of the epithelium is anything but atrophic. In fact, epithelial proliferation in all forms of chronic gastritis is increased, and the zone of proliferating cells appears to be expanded. This may be of importance with regard to the malignant predisposition of these conditions (see Section 5).

Gastric mucosal epithelial proliferation has also been shown to be increased in Z–E syndrome. Serum gastrin levels are markedly elevated in Z–E syndrome. Similarly, serum gastrin levels may be elevated in chronic gastritis as a consequence of parietal cell dropout and hyposecretion of acid. Thus, the stimulation of epithelial proliferation in both Z–E syndrome and chronic gastritis, which differ dramatically in clinical manifestations, is in keeping with the known trophic effects of gastrin on the gastric mucosa.

Information about epithelial proliferation in peptic disease of the duodenum is limited. Autoradiographic studies of biopsies from patients with duodenal ulcers or nonulcer duodenitis show that proliferation is increased in the inflamed mucosa adjacent to active ulcers and in duodenitis, when compared with normal-appearing mucosa from control subjects without peptic disease. Furthermore, proliferation in histological normal biopsies from sites removed from active ulceration in the ulcer patients is normal. Thus, epithelial proliferation in duodenal ulcer disease does not appear to be impaired.

5. RELEVANCE OF ABNORMALITIES IN EPITHELIAL RENEWAL TO CARCINOGENESIS

Abnormal epithelial renewal, that is, an increase in numbers of proliferating cells and expansion of the proliferative zone, has been associated with frank neoplasia and a number of so-called premalignant conditions of the GI tract. In the upper GI tract, these conditions include Barrett's epithelium, intestinal metaplasia of the stomach, and chronic gastritis. In the large bowel, similar abnormalities have been described in ulcerative colitis and histologically normal colonic mucosa throughout the colon of patients with polyps or cancers. In fact, some relatives of patients with colonic neoplasms also have abnormal proliferation kinetics. Interesting recent work indicates that oral calcium supplementation, in doses of about 1200–1500 mg/day, reverses these abnormalities in the colon.

Moreover, in a large population study, high dietary calcium intake appeared to be related to a low risk of developing colon cancer. Other agents, such as vitamin C, also appear to reverse the abnormal pattern of proliferation and, in experimental animals, decrease the yield of expected tumors after administration of the potent carcinogen, dimethylhydrazine. Whether therapeutic normalization of premalignant patterns of epithelial proliferation will lead to a reduction in tumor development remains to be shown. However, it is tempting to speculate that in years to come we will be treating our patients who have Barrett's epithelium and other premalignant conditions with such ordinary supplements as calcium and vitamin C.

6. CONCLUSIONS: RELEVANCE OF ABNORMALITIES IN EPITHELIAL CELL RENEWAL TO CYTOPROTECTION

The concept of cytoprotection has evolved to include virtually any mechanism whereby the mucosa of the esophagus, stomach, or duodenum can be protected against injury. It is inherently clear that an intact functional epithelial lining of the upper GI tract is of critical importance in maintaining the integrity of the mucosa. Furthermore, epithelial cells are responsible for the secretion of mucus, bicarbonate, and the phospholipid layer that adheres to their apical surfaces, all of which are believed to be important mechanisms of mucosal protection. Thus, it is reasonable to propose that agents or conditions that inhibit epithelial renewal in the upper GI tract predispose to mucosal injury either by retarding the healing of existing mucosal lesions or by accelerating the formation of new ones. The inhibiting effects of corticosteroids and of stress on gastric antral and fundic epithelial proliferation and the failure of antral epithelial proliferation to respond to aspirin or indomethacin may be clinically relevant examples of the importance of alterations in epithelial renewal in the pathogenesis of mucosal injury.

Is it possible to use our knowledge of the regulation of epithelial renewal to therapeutic advantage? Certainly, it makes good sense to avoid agents or conditions that interfere with the process of epithelial renewal when we can. But we already know that aspirin, stress, and corticosteroids are not necessarily good for patients. Currently available therapeutic agents, such as acid-inhibiting and mucosal cytoprotective drugs, in addition to their other beneficial effects, create an environment in which the process of epithelial renewal can take place. However, active intervention to control one or more aspects of epithelial renewal is not yet part of the therapeutic strategy. This could take the form of stimulation of epithelial proliferation or, perhaps, retardation of epithelial cell loss. Certain agents, such as gastrin, are known to be trophic to gastric fundic and duodenal epithelium. However, gastrin would not be an appropriate therapeutic agent because of its stimulatory effects on acid secretion. Prostaglandin administration is associated with a thickening of the gastric mucosa, which does not appear to be caused by stimulation of epithelial proliferation but rather by inhibition of cell loss. Thus, in addition to their other beneficial effects, prostaglandins may promote cytoprotection by regulating the rate of epithelial cell loss.

Can we augment in some manner the process of restitution, whereby the rapid migration of epithelial cells heals areas of mild mucosal surface injury? Would stimulation of epithelial proliferation be a useful adjunct in the treatment of peptic disease? Clearly this ground is fertile for future research.

ANNOTATED BIBLIOGRAPHY

Bizzozero G: Uber die Regeneration der Elemente der schlauchformigen Drusen und des Epithels des Magendarmkanals. *Anat Anz* **3:**781–784, 1888.

Original prediction of epithelial renewal based on the observation of mitotic figures identified by light microscopy.

Eastwood GL: Gastrointestinal epithelial renewal. *Gastroenterology* **72:**962–975, 1977.

General review of gastrointestinal epithelial renewal.

Eastwood GL, Kuwayama H: Effects of ulcerogens and other conditions on gastric epithelial proliferation, in Szabo S, Pfeiffer C (eds): *Ulcer Disease: New Aspects of Pathogenesis and Pharmacology.* Boca Raton, FL, CRC Press, 1989.

Details of the studies of the effects of aspirin, indomethacin, alcohol, histamine-2 antagonists, steroids, and water immersion restraint stress on epithelial proliferation.

Garland C, Shekelle RB, Barrett-Connor E, et al: Dietary vitamin D and calcium and risk of colorectal cancer: A 19-year prospective study in men. *Lancet* **1:**307–309, 1985.

Epidemiological study showing a decreased risk of colon cancer associated with high dietary calcium.

Ito S, Lacy ER: Morphology of rat gastric mucosal damage, defense, and restitution in the presence of luminal ethanol. *Gastroenterology* **88:**250–260, 1985.

Description of the process of restitution.

Lipkin M: Growth and development of gastrointestinal cells. *Annu Rev Physiol* **47:**175–197, 1985.

Review of gastrointestinal epithelial renewal, with an emphasis on recent developments in experimental methods to study proliferation and differentiation.

Lipkin M, Newmark H: Effect of added dietary calcium on colonic epithelial-cell proliferation in subjects at high risk for familial colonic cancer. *N Engl J Med* **313:**1381–1383, 1985.

Dietary calcium normalizes the abnormal epithelial proliferation in rectal biopsies from relatives of patients with colon cancer.

McNeil NO, Eikenburg BE, Johnson LR: Role of ornithine decarboxylase in functional development of rat gastric mucosa. *Am J Physiol* **252**:G466–G471, 1987.

Description of the role of the polyamines, putrescine, spermidine, and spermine, and of the enzyme, ornithine decarboxylase (ODC), in epithelial proliferation.

8

Gastric Blood Flow and Mucosal Defense

PETER J. OATES

1. INTRODUCTION

Any other tissue would rapidly disintegrate if exposed to the corrosive acid that bathes the lining of the stomach. The gastric lining, or mucosa, also resists all but the harshest of miscellaneous chemical insults. It is no surprise, then, that this tissue has intrigued doctors and scientists for centuries, particularly with regard to how it achieves such remarkable Teflon-like chemical resistance properties. It is only relatively recently, however, that the defensive secrets of the gastric mucosa have begun to be appreciated in detail. This chapter describes one of the central elements of the gastric mucosal defensive system, blood flow. It is recognized that blood flow is also pivotal to mucosal restitution and the healing processes. However, the emphasis here is on the role of mucosal blood flow in preventing the initiation of gastric lesions. The reader will also note that other important components of the gastric defensive system are covered in substantial depth in other chapters of this volume. For this reason, only very brief mention of these other important defensive factors will be made here.

2. THE GASTRIC VASCULATURE

The vascular system of the stomach constitutes a superb example of the integration of biological structure and function. The general anatomical design of the gastric vasculature and its functional implications is briefly reviewed.

PETER J. OATES • Central Research Division, Pfizer Inc., Department of Metabolic Diseases, Groton, Connecticut 06340.

2.1. General Anatomical Design

2.1.1. Arterial Supply

The arterial supply of the stomach originates in one of the major branches of the abdominal aorta, the celiac artery (Fig. 1). As shown schematically in Fig. 1, the stomach is perfused by at least six different major arteries or arterial groups: the right and left gastric, the right and left gastroepiploic, and the short branches of the splenic and of the gastroduodenal arteries. In addition to these, very often there are six secondary arteries supplying the stomach. Anastomosis occurs freely among the 12 vessels. Indeed, extensive anastomosis is perhaps the most striking design feature of gross gastric vascular anatomy. For example, note the continuity of the right and left gastric and of the right and left gastroepiploic arteries in Fig. 1. This key design feature extends down to the small vessels within the gastric wall. As shown schematically in Fig. 2, external gastric arteries enter the gastric wall through the external muscle layer, the muscularis. As, and after, the arteries pass through the muscularis, they give off arterioles that supply the capillary beds of the muscularis. On entering the loose connective tissue of the submucosa, the small gastric arteries branch and anastomose, forming a submucosal network or plexus (Fig. 2). The small gastric arteries or arterial plexi give rise to adrenergically innervated submucosal arterioles. The arterioles pass into and through the muscularis mucosa (Fig. 2), where they branch into terminal mucosal arterioles that subdivide into mucosal capillaries.

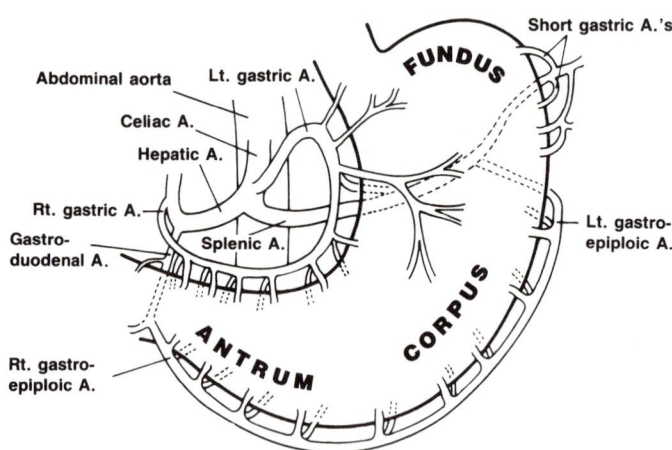

Figure 1. Major arterial supply of the human stomach. (Modified from Guth and Leung, 1987.)

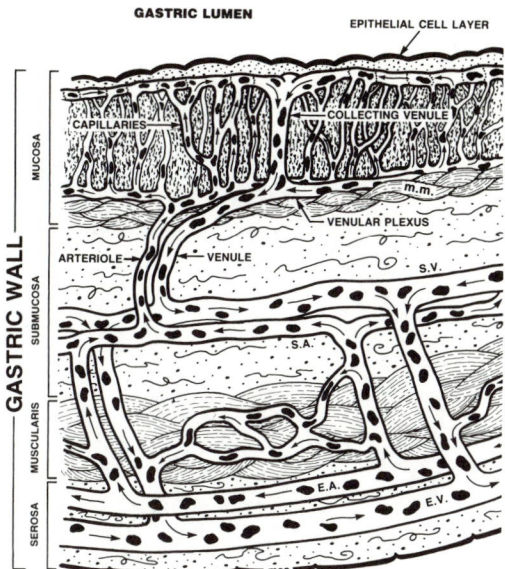

Figure 2. Schematic structure of the vasculature of the gastric wall. Significant species differences in gastric vascular architecture have not been reported among mammals. The vascular structure immediately beneath the epithelial cell layer (drawn containing dotted lines), represents a side view of the superficial polygonal vascular network shown en face in Fig. 3A. The tubular gastric glands are omitted in Fig. 2 for clarity. EA, external artery; EV, external vein; mes, mesothelium; mm, muscularis mucosa; SA, submucosal artery; SV, submucosal vein.

2.1.2. Mucosal Capillaries

At the very bottom of the glandular mucosa, mucosal capillaries sprout from the terminal arterioles and generally run perpendicularly up around the tubular gastric glands, packed like test tubes in the mucosa (Figs. 2 and 3A). Precapillary sphincters have not been clearly demonstrated in mucosal capillaries. As the capillaries traverse the mucosa, they interconnect horizontally (Fig. 2) to form a vascular lacework around the gastric glands. Important ultrastructural features of mucosal capillaries are that their walls are thin and are fenestrated, i.e., the endothelial cells that constitute their walls have numerous small windowlike thin spots. Such capillaries are typically found in the tissue zones of relatively high permeability to hydrophilic solutes. The observation that the protein concentration in gastric lymph is as high as 50% that of plasma reinforces the notion that mucosal capillaries are highly permeable. Individual capillaries that run up through the thickness of the mucosa connect into a superficial polygonal vascular network located just beneath the one-cell-thick epithelial layer (Figs. 2 and 3). This superficial bed of capillaries and postcapillary venules forms an essentially two-dimensional honeycomblike network parallel to the mucosal surface. Each superficial vascular polygon in the network forms a collar around the superficial end of a tubular gastric gland (GG) (Fig. 3A, B). Thus, centered over each

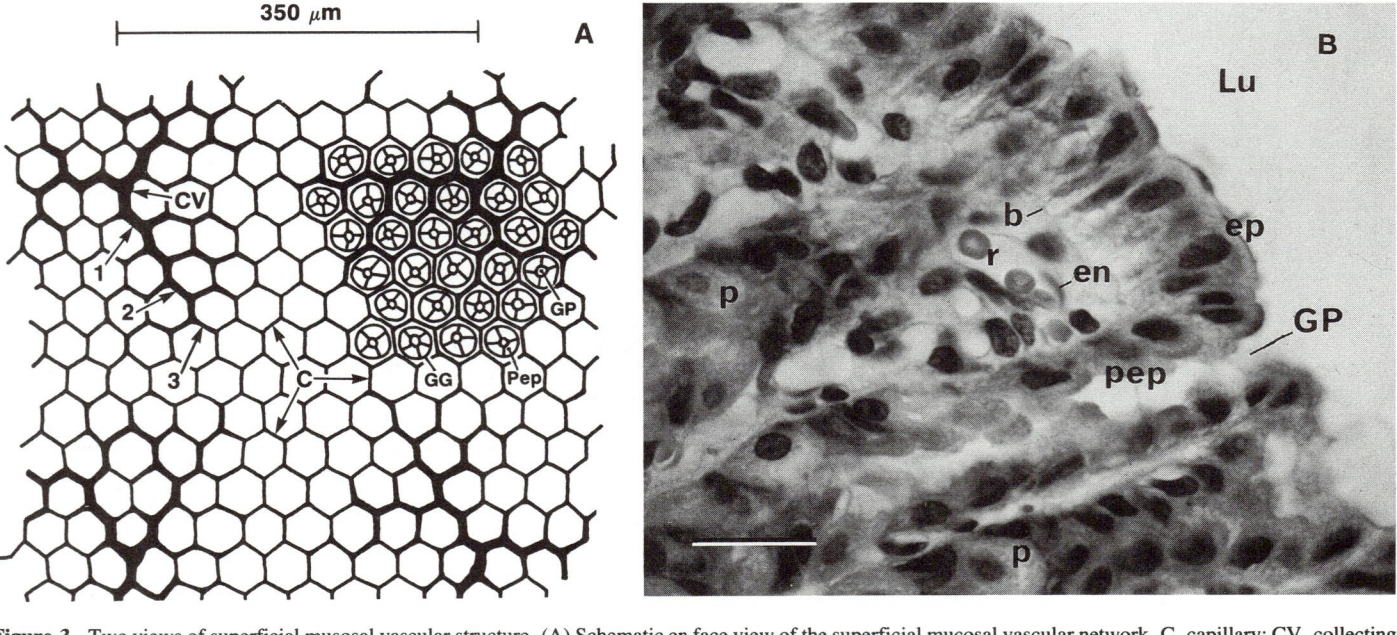

Figure 3. Two views of superficial musosal vascular structure. (A) Schematic en face view of the superficial mucosal vascular network. C, capillary; CV, collecting venule; 1, 2, 3, first-, second-, and third-order postcapillary venule, respectively; GG, gastric gland (cross section); GP, gastric pit; pep, pit epithelial cell. (Modified from Holm-Rutili and Öbrink, 1985.) (B) Histological section of normal rat stomach cut approximately perpendicularly to the mucosal surface. Elements of the superficial vascular network are seen in cross section as erythrocyte (r)-containing spaces bounded by endothelial cells (en). b, basement membrane; ep, epithelial cells; Lu, gastric lumen; p, parietal cells; other labels as in A. (H & E stain; bar = 20 μm.)

vascular polygon, the lumen or gastric pit (GP) of each individual GG communicates with the gastric lumen (Lu).

2.1.3. Venous Pattern

On entering the superficial vascular network from the mucosal capillaries, blood sweeps under the epithelial surface through capillary vessels, which enlarge to become small superficial venular elements that lead into collecting venules (Figs. 2 and 3). Although uniformly distributed, these oak tree-like venules are comparatively infrequent (Figs 2 and 3A). They are larger in diameter and thicker walled than mucosal capillaries. Mucosal collecting venules are not fenestrated and are surrounded by a significantly thicker layer of connective tissue than are mucosal capillaries. Collecting venules receive little or no venular tributaries once they begin their descent through the mucosa (Fig. 2). Collecting venules run essentially perpendicularly downward from the mucosal surface to a venular plexus at the bottom of the mucosa. The deep mucosal venular plexus is drained by submucosal venules that generally follow quite closely the pattern of submucosal arterial vessels (Fig. 4). The submucosal venules lead into small submucosal veins that also tend to follow closely the small arteries, back up through the external muscle to connect with external gastric veins (Figs. 2 and 4). As the gastric veins pass through the muscularis, they receive small venules that drain the muscle (Fig. 2). Intramural and external gastric veins do not have valves. They exhibit adrenergic innervation, but it is limited relative to that of the arterioles and small arteries. Contrary to some earlier reports, most recent studies have failed to demonstrate arteriovenous shunts in human or animal gastric tissue. However, controversy still lingers around this topic.

2.2. Functional Implications

The vascular structure just described carries a number of implications about the fundamental functional properties of the stomach and of mucosal blood flow.

2.2.1. Resistance to Focal Arterial Occlusion

Blood flow is a vital part of the defense of the gastric mucosa against luminal acid. Unchecked, luminal acid can cause perforation of the gastric wall, severe hemorrhage, and death. Were blood flow to a zone of the mucosa vulnerable to an embolus lodging in a particular artery, the consequences could thus be lethal. However, the extensive network of vascular anastomoses throughout the

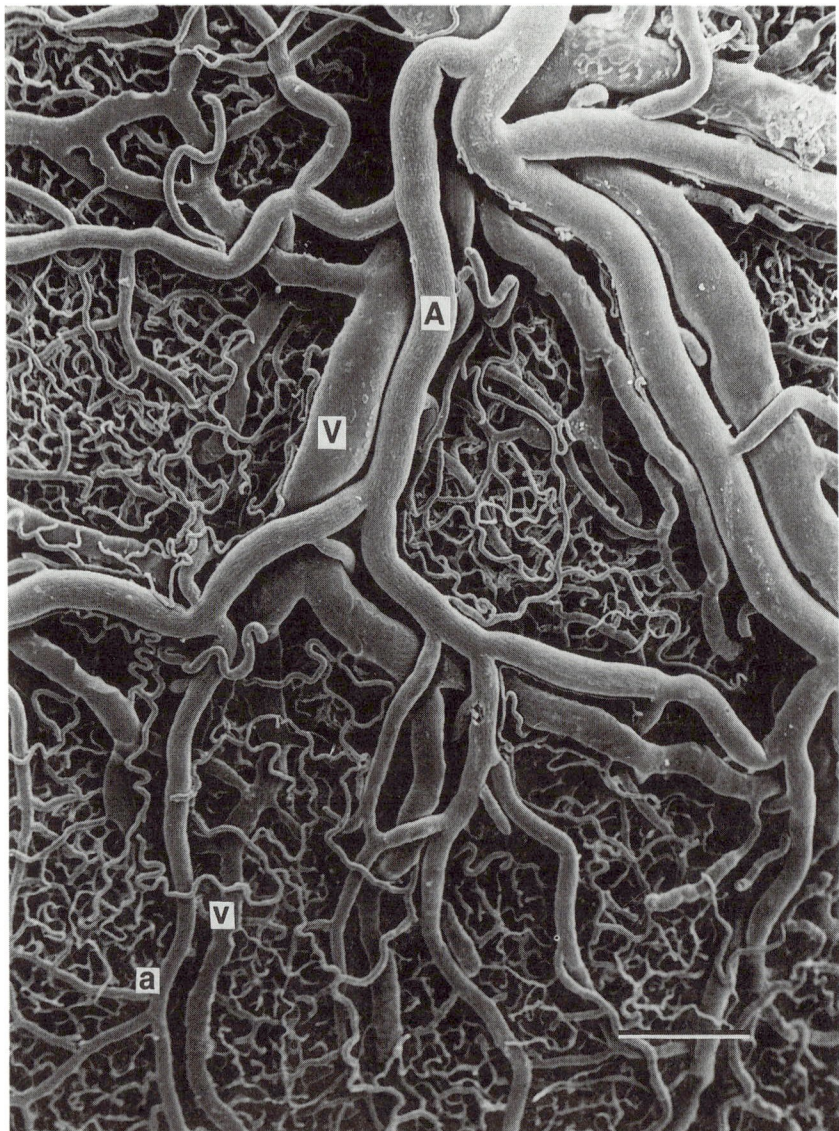

Figure 4. Arterial and venous vessels of the gastric submucosa. Note the proximity of submucosal veins (V) to arteries (A) and of venules (v) to arterioles (a). The very small-diameter vessels are deep mucosal capillaries. Bar = 300 μm. (From Gannon *et al.*, 1982.)

stomach wall makes the wall extremely resistant to instances of arterial occlusion. The lack of valves in intramural gastric veins provides additional insurance by allowing reverse blood flow to aid potentially jeopardized tissue zones. The overall point is well illustrated by the fact that some 90% of the arterial supply of the canine stomach must be ligated before gastric blood flow is significantly compromised.

2.2.2. Functional Implications

Extensive vascular anastomoses help ensure an uninterrupted blood supply to the stomach lining. However, to achieve efficient local control of blood flow, nonanastomosing bottlenecks in the arterial network are needed. These are provided by the submucosal arterioles and small postplexus submucosal arteries (Figs. 2 and 4). Rich adrenergic innervation of these vessels also indicates that they are regulatory sites. Moreover, it has been observed experimentally that dilation of submucosal arterioles results in increased flow velocity in the superficial mucosal vascular network. Conversely, constriction of submucosal arterioles causes reduced superficial mucosal flow. Thus, a major factor controlling local mucosal flow is the diameter of submucosal arterioles. As in other tissue beds, the slightly larger prearteriolar arteries probably also contribute to flow control.

2.2.3. Site of Relative Restriction of Superficial Flow

The anatomical structure of the superficial vascular network also has important functional implications. As blood moves through the superficial network from a capillary (C) to a collecting venule (CV) (see Fig. 3A), the diameters of the blood vessels enlarge by a factor of approximately 2 (Table I). Flow velocity does not drop; rather, it increases in conjunction with the blood being carried by increasingly fewer vessels as the collecting venule is approached (Fig. 3a; Table I). Since flow is the product of vessel luminal cross-sectional area and flow velocity, blood flow through different segments of the superficial vascular network therefore varies markedly. The capillary portions of the superficial vascular network have the smallest diameter, the slowest flow velocity, and the lowest rate of blood flow (Table I). Compared with the next smallest size segment, the third-order venule, blood flow in capillary segments is two to three times less. Compared with the largest size segment, the first order venule, blood flow in capillary segments is $15\times$ less (Table I). Thus, a distinct gradient of blood flow occurs within the superficial mucosal vascular network, as suggested

Table I. Blood Flow in the Superficial Vascular Network of Rat Mucosa[a]

	Order of venular vessels[b]			
	1st	2nd	3rd	Capillaries
Diameter (μm)	14.5[c]	10.0[d]	7.9[f]	6.5
	±0.54	±0.37	±0.54	±0.38
V_{RBC} (mm/sec)	0.43	0.28[d]	0.25	0.15[d]
	±0.03	±0.02	±0.04	±0.01
Volume flow (ml/sec)	0.075	0.024[d]	0.013[e]	0.005[d]
	±0.0074	±0.0024	±0.0026	±0.0008
N	36	28	13	8

[a]From Holm-Rutili and Öbrink (1985).
[b]Refer to Fig. 3A.
[c]Values are means ±SEM; N, no. of animals. V_{RBC}, red blood cell velocity.
[d]$p < 0.001$.
[e]$p < 0.01$.
[f]$p < .05$ compared with the next larger vessel.

by Fig. 3A and the data in Table I. Since blood flow through this network constitutes a critical element of the gastric mucosal barrier, these quantitative focal differences in superficial flow become important when luminal acid probes the relative barrier function at different areas of the mucosal surface. That is, other things being equal, barrier function will be weakest at mucosal zones overlying areas of lowest blood flow, i.e., overlying capillaries at points midway between collecting venules (Fig. 3A). This zone of relatively weak barrier function is the preferential initiation site of certain types of acid-dependent mucosal lesions (see Section 5.1.1).

2.2.4. Upward Intramucosal Flow Pattern

Mucosal arterial blood flows from the bottom of the mucosa up to the luminal surface, flowing by way of numerous mucosal capillaries oriented essentially perpendicularly to the mucosal surface (Fig. 2). These capillaries, which are thin-walled, fenestrated, and of relatively high surface area to volume, are clearly designed for efficient molecular exchange with the nearby metabolically active cells of the gastric glands. However, this is not the case for the 30- to 50-μm diameter collecting venules that carry blood downward, away from the mucosal surface (see Fig. 2). Based simply on cylindrical vessel diameters, a 40-μm collecting venule has a surface area-to-volume ratio some six times smaller than that of a 6.5-μm capillary. When the relative numbers of the two types of mucosal vessels are considered, the difference is further magnified. Each collecting venule in the rat mucosa drains approximately 60 gastric pits, which are estimated to be supported by a total of roughly 100 vertical mucosal capillaries (see Fig. 3A). Human mucosa appears quite similar. Mucosal capillaries thus present a relative surface area available for exchange with the mucosal interstitium that is some 16 times greater than that of the collecting venules. Put differently, mucosal capillaries can be estimated to constitute some 94% of the total vascular surface area available for solute exchange within the mucosa. Furthermore, when it is recalled that the endothelial wall of the collecting venule is relatively thick, is not fenestrated, and is surrounded by a relatively thick connective tissue layer, it is clear that mucosal collecting venules are designed to function like raingutter downspouts on a house, i.e., they are essentially one-way transport vessels. Thus, diffusional molecular movements and exchange within the mucosa are totally dominated by upward convection rooted in unidirectional capillary flow. This architecturally mediated reversed fountain flow pattern is an important component of the mucosal barrier and has important implications for mucosal function.

2.2.5. Venous–Arterial Feedback?

Local regulation of blood flow is widely believed to occur in part by diffusional feedback of vasoactive products of cell metabolism. For example, if perfusion of cardiac tissue with oxygenated blood becomes insufficient relative to local metabolic demand, vasodilatory metabolites such as adenosine are released from cardiac cells. Adenosine diffuses to small arteries and arterioles and causes dilation, thereby increasing local blood flow to match the local need. In the gastric mucosa, however, such a mechanism seemingly encounters a serious logistical difficulty because of the upward blood flow pattern discussed in Section 2.2.4. That is, vasodilatory metabolites generated in mucosal tissue as feedback signals will be physically unable to diffuse directly back to the flow-controlling arterioles and small arteries. Instead, they will be swept up to the mucosal surface and carried down through the mucosal collecting venules to the deep mucosal and submucosal venular plexi (see Fig. 2).

A possible solution to this problem lies in postulating that local feedback regulation of arteriolar and small artery tone occurs directly or indirectly across the venular walls adjacent to submucosal arterial vessels (see Figs. 2 and 4). There is little to prevent low-molecular-weight vasoregulatory substances from crossing deep mucosal or submucosal venular walls, especially gases such as nitrous oxide (N_2O) or carbon dioxide (CO_2). Moreover, the permeability of venules is well known to be enhanced by vasoactive substances such as histamine, which also dilates submucosal arterioles. Both histamine and vasodilatory prostaglandins occur in greater amounts in gastric venous blood than in gastric arterial blood. This indicates that these substances are produced by mucosal tissue and diffuse into the gastric venular system. Such vasoregulatory substances or secondarily generated mediators could act directly on the smooth muscle of arterial resistance vessels in the immediate vicinity (see Fig. 4) or possibly on vascular nerves, or both. Such a feedback loop would appear to provide a rapid and efficient way for the metabolic status of the overlying mucosa to be responsively monitored by the underlying arterial vessels. This concept thus implies that the intimate association of small arterial and venous vessels observed in the gastric mucosa (see Fig. 4), as well as in many other vascular beds, might represent much more than mere plumbing convenience. However, until this concept is examined experimentally, it must remain hypothetical.

3. PHYSIOLOGICAL REGULATION OF MUCOSAL BLOOD FLOW

3.1. Basal Flow

As in any other vascular bed, gastric blood flow is regulated by a combination of nervous and humoral factors. The principal ones are diagrammatically indicated in Fig. 5. Basal mucosal blood flow appears to reflect a balance between sympathetic adrenergic vasoconstriction versus metabolite- and/or autocoid-mediated vasodilation. The identities of the primary vasodilatory substances controlling basal mucosal blood flow are unclear. Leading possibilities include histamine, prostaglandins, adenosine, CO_2, or protons. Basal flow also appears to be linked to intramucosal pH regulation (see Section 4.3.3). Under basal conditions, about 80–90% of the total gastric flow is to the mucosa–submucosa and about 75% is to the mucosa. One important feature of gastric blood flow is that it varies directly with mean arterial pressure (Fig. 5). Thus, in contrast to certain tissues, such as the kidney, the stomach does not autoregulate; i.e., when a change in arterial pressure occurs, the stomach does not try to maintain constant flow via a compensatory change in its vascular resistance. This basic characteristic of gastric tissue has important pathophysiological implications (see Section 5.1).

3.2. Stimulated Flow

When gastric secretion is stimulated by neural or chemical means, total gastric blood flow increases severalfold. Most of the increased flow is to the

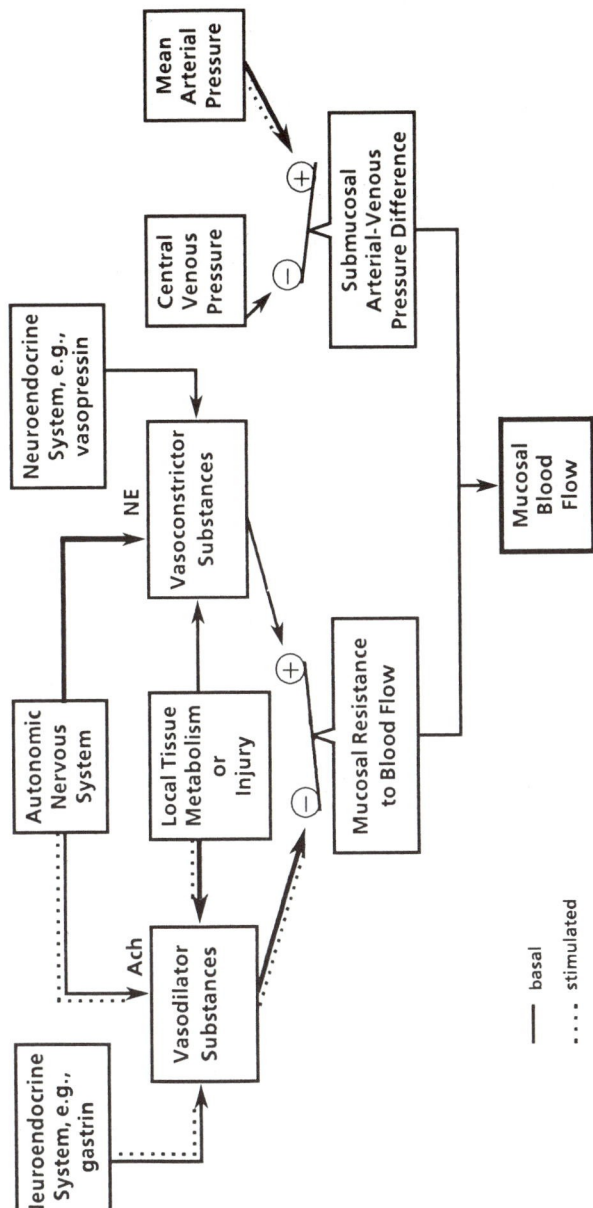

Figure 5. Basic factors that determine mucosal blood flow. Predominant factors under basal conditions (—); major influences under stimulated conditions (....).

mucosa. The increased flow provides oxygen and nutrients to support the intensely energy-demanding work of acid, mucus, bicarbonate, and pepsin secretion. Enhanced blood flow is also important in helping the mucosa defend itself against its own highly acidic secretion. The identities of the mediators of physiologically stimulated mucosal blood flow are poorly defined. In addition to the possible mediators mentioned in connection with basal flow, additional mediators for stimulated flow include acetylcholine (ACh) and neuroendocrine substances. Inhibition of stimulated gastric secretion causes a corresponding drop in stimulated mucosal blood flow. However, under some conditions, these two variables can be dissociated. The recent availability of new pharmacological tools, e.g., proton pump inhibitors and high-affinity histamine H_2-antagonists, should promote a better understanding of the mechanisms involved in regulating basal and stimulated mucosal blood flow.

4. BLOOD FLOW AND THE GASTRIC MUCOSAL BARRIER

4.1. The Mucosal Barrier

The lining of the stomach is remarkably resilient. Even when drastic topical challenges, such as concentrated acid, base, or alcohol, are used to produce gross injury to normal mucosa, the incidence of lesion formation is often less than 100%. This surprising resistance to gross injury is attributable to the so-called gastric mucosal barrier. The barrier is not a particular structural entity. It is a very sophisticated multicomponent system that ordinarily permits mucosal tissue to reside comfortably in contact with highly corrosive HCl. Although pepsin, the protease of gastric juice, can contribute to tissue damage once the barrier has been breached, most investigators do not consider pepsin a significant aggressive factor in initiating mucosal damage. This is because the relatively large molecular size of pepsin hinders it from penetrating surface mucus, and therefore from contacting the mucosal surface. Moreover, the proteolytic activity of pepsin is dependent on very low pH, a circumstance that may not pertain in the microenvironment of the alkali-secreting surface epithelial cells.

Thus, HCl is considered the major aggressive factor initiating mucosal damage; the gastric mucosal barrier has increasingly become conceptualized as that combination of factors that enables the mucosa to prevent tissue acidification. The various components of the barrier are described in some detail in earlier chapters. In the present case, a brief summary of barrier structure and function will be given, emphasizing the central role played by mucosal blood flow.

4.2. Nonvascular Barrier Components

The major components of the barrier include mucus, phospholipids, bicarbonate, epithelial cell plasma membranes, cell-to-cell tight junctions, and a bicarbonate-rich blood supply (Fig. 6). Mucosal mast cells (mc) also constitute part of the barrier. Under some pathophysiological circumstances, these cells play an important role in barrier function; this may also be the case under ordinary physiological conditions (see Section 4.4).

Barrier components function in concert to limit the diffusion of protons down a very strong lumen-to-tissue chemical concentration gradient, some 3,000,000 : 1. The major structural feature that limits the leakage of hydrogen ions into the mucosa appears to be the surface epithelial cell layer itself. Surface epithelial cells defend themselves with an armament of ion pumps and ion exchangers, with intracellular and extracellular bicarbonate, and with secreted mucus (e.g., see Chapters 5 and 6). The mucus appears to be rich in a particular species of phospholipid, dipalmitoylphosphatidylcholine, better known as pulmonary surfactant. Gastric mucus has also been found to contain covalently bound fatty acids. The presence of these fatty substances adds a waxlike hydrophobic character to the mucosal surface that may also confer a protective effect from hydrophilic substances. The basement membranes provide structural support for the epithelial cells tethered to them, but basement membranes are not known to constitute a barrier to small ion traffic.

Influxing protons are normally rapidly neutralized by subepithelial interstitial bicarbonate. When monitored with a pH-sensitive microelectrode whose tip was positioned 10–30 μm below rat mucosal epithelium, a slight relative acidification (~pH 6.9–7.1 versus ~pH 7.25–7.35) was detected with 100–150 mM luminal HCl compared with luminal saline. How much deeper into the

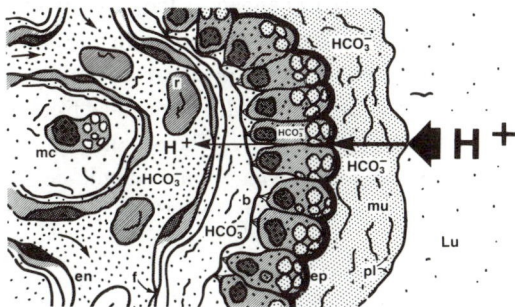

Figure 6. Major components of the gastric mucosal barrier. b, basement membrane; en, endothelial cells; ep, epithelial cells; f, fenestrations; H^+, protons; HCO_3^-, bicarbonate; Lu, gastric lumen; mc, mucosal mast cell; mu, mucus; pl, phospholipid; r, red blood cell.

mucosa this relative acidification is detectable is unknown. Its absence at the midpoint of mucosal thickness suggests that, under normal circumstances, probably not very far.

4.3. Role of Blood Flow in Barrier Function

4.3.1. Bicarbonate and Nutrient Transport

Mucosal blood flow supports the defensive mechanisms mentioned above by supplying oxygen and fuel to the mucosal cells involved in maintaining the transepithelial barrier to HCl. Blood flow also removes metabolic wastes and CO_2 resulting from mucosal metabolism and from neutralization of influxing acid. In addition, mucosal blood flow is critically important in helping control intratissue pH, because it is the vehicle by which bicarbonate is transported into the superficial mucosa and by which excess protons are removed from the tissue.

Blood-borne mucosal bicarbonate comes largely from two sources. First, during acid secretion, copious quantities of bicarbonate are generated locally by upstream gastric parietal cells located just a short distance below the superficial epithelium. As the parietal cells secrete protons across their apical surface, they simultaneously secrete bicarbonate across their basolateral surfaces. The bicarbonate readily diffuses into the fenestrated mucosal capillaries located adjacent to the basal surface of the parietal cells. The upward flow of capillary blood transports the bicarbonate up into the superficial polygonal vascular network underlying the epithelial cell layer. From there, bicarbonate can diffuse into the superficial interstitium, and reach the basal aspect of the epithelium (Fig. 6). Besides directly neutralizing penetrating protons, interstitial bicarbonate may be transported into mucosal cells for intracellular buffering and for local secretion. The availability of bicarbonate clearly enhances the capacity of mucosal cells to resist damage. Gastric parietal cells provide a very rich source of bicarbonate, as evidenced by the occurrence of the well-known alkaline tide that accompanies gastric secretion. That is, enough bicarbonate is generated from secreting parietal cells to raise gastric venous pH detectably. The second source of blood-borne bicarbonate is the systemic pool derived from systemic cell metabolism and respiration. This provides a large reservoir of bicarbonate under basal conditions.

4.3.2. Proton and Xenobiotic Transport

Blood flow also plays an important protective role by physically diluting and removing nonneutralized protons from superficial mucosal tissue. This function becomes prominent when blood-borne bicarbonate becomes saturated or when exogenous irritating chemicals other than acid (xenobiotics) penetrate the superficial mucosa. In the latter case, blood flow can also serve to deliver the xenobiotic to the liver via the portal circulation for detoxification or excretion or both, thus reducing subsequent tissue exposure of all organs, including the gastric mucosa, to the xenobiotic.

4.3.3. Regulation of Intramucosal pH

Under normal physiological conditions, the ultimate functional objective of the gastric mucosal barrier is to defend interstitial pH to the degree necessary to prevent the intracellular pH regulatory systems of mucosal cells from being overwhelmed. Although the cellular mechanisms for regulating cytoplasmic pH are efficient, they are basically low-capacity systems designed for local fine-tuning and can be relatively easily saturated by the very strong pH gradients potentially arising in mucosal tissue. Thus, preventing cell death from cytoplasmic acidification depends on effectively regulating intracellular pH. This, in turn, requires maintaining a relatively constant extracellular (interstitial) pH, or at least a level at which changes capable of exceeding cellular regulatory capacities do not occur.

The factors that determine mucosal interstitial pH are diagrammatically summarized in Fig. 7. The interstitial hydrogen ion concentration $[H^+]$ can be viewed as the sum of any arbitrarily chosen preceding value of interstitial hydrogen ion concentration $[H^+]_0$ plus any change (positive or negative) in interstitial hydrogen concentration $\Delta[H^+]$, that has occurred over the arbitrarily chosen time interval examined:

$$[H^+] = [H^+]_0 + \Delta[H^+]$$

Any change in interstitial hydrogen ion concentration $\Delta[H^+]$ is equal to the difference between total interstitial proton influx and total interstitial proton efflux (the latter term including chemical efflux, i.e., neutralization) (Fig. 7). Total interstitial proton efflux is critically dependent on mucosal blood flow. Again, mucosal blood flow is needed to deliver bicarbonate for neutralization reactions and to remove physically any excess protons.

Little is known about the regulation of interstitial pH. Several observations indicate that intramucosal pH is regulated and that mucosal blood flow plays a central role in the regulatory system. For example, if the mucosal surface is damaged by acidified bile salt, an abnormally high amount of acid enters into the superficial mucosa; the barrier has been broken. However, the tissue does not

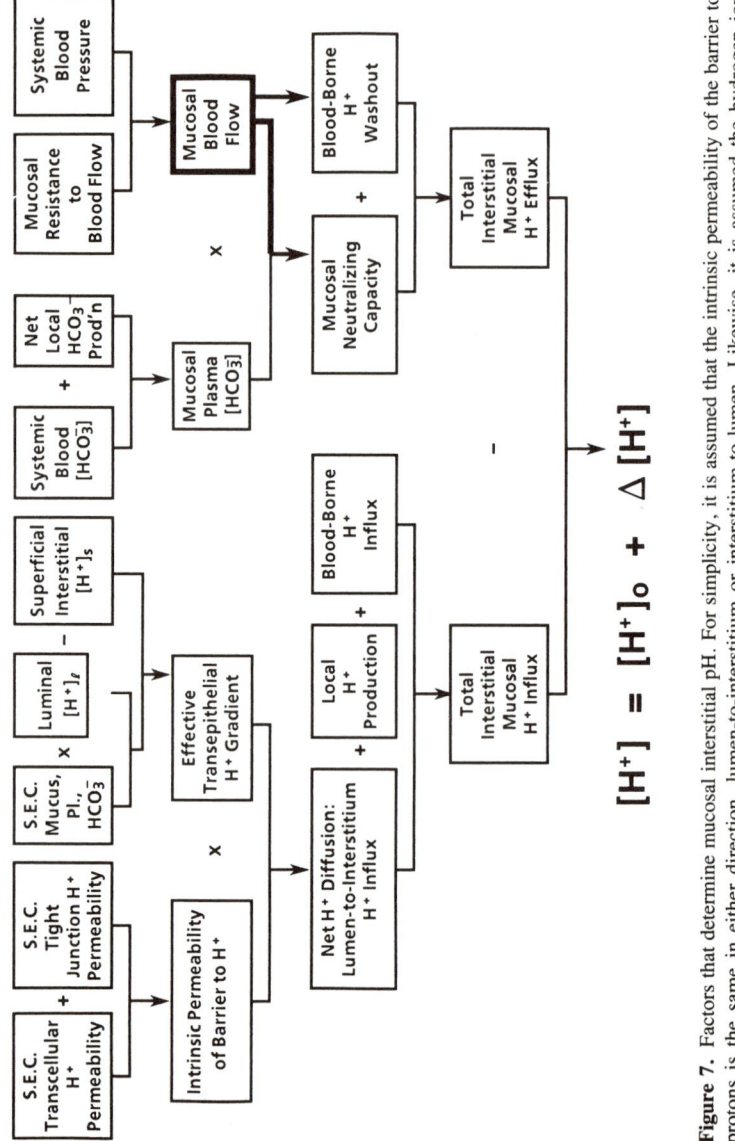

Figure 7. Factors that determine mucosal interstitial pH. For simplicity, it is assumed that the intrinsic permeability of the barrier to protons is the same in either direction, lumen-to-interstitium or interstitium-to-lumen. Likewise, it is assumed the hydrogen ion concentration in the gastric lumen, $[H^+]_l$, is much greater than the hydrogen ion concentration in the superficial interstitium, $[H^+]_s$. The net H^+ diffusional movement will therefore be a lumen-to-interstitial influx. S.E.C., superficial epithelial cell; Pl., phospholipid; $[H^+]$, interstitial hydrogen ion concentration; $[H^+]_o$, interstitial hydrogen ion concentration at any preceding time; $\Delta[H^+]$, the change in interstitial hydrogen ion concentration since $[H^+]_o$.

become significantly damaged because the mucosa responds by increasing mucosal blood flow in direct proportion to the abnormal excess of incoming acid (Fig. 8). This is apparently associated with the intramural pH remaining virtually constant (see Section 5.1.1). By contrast, raising the pH of mucosal blood is reported to cause a decrease in mucosal blood flow.

Thus, it seems that basal mucosal blood flow is adjusted as necessary to maintain constant mucosal pH. This implies the existence of a blood flow-linked mucosal system for regulating mucosal pH. This hypothetical system is referred to here as the mucosal pH-stat system (Fig. 9). It is hypothesized to consist of the mucosal vasculature and those elements necessary to monitor and control mucosal pH by means of regulation of mucosal blood flow. Key among these elements is a pH-stat, i.e., an element that senses the local pH, compares it with a predetermined setpoint, and directly or indirectly causes an increased release of one or more vasodilatory mediators. The resulting enhanced mucosal blood flow and bicarbonate delivery bring the superficial pH back toward (or, if local bicarbonate secretion has been activated, even temporarily past) the normal setpoint.

Thus, as suggested in Fig. 9, one way to view the gastric mucosal barrier is that it consists of two major functional units, a largely structural coarse filter, and a largely functional blood flow-linked pH-stat system. The coarse filter corresponds to the epithelial cell layer with its covering of alkaline fatty mucus. The coarse filter reduces the rate of proton influx into the mucosa by orders of magnitude, down to a range that can be efficiently dealt with by the readily adjustable mucosal pH-stat system.

It must be emphasized that critical experimental testing of this pH-stat concept has yet to be done. The upper and lower limits of the regulated range

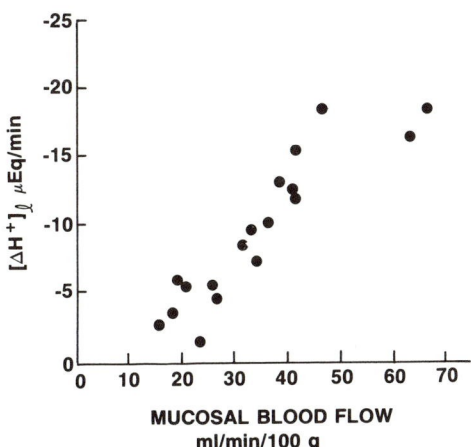

Figure 8. Relationship between net luminal H^+ loss, $\Delta[H^+]_l$, and mucosal blood flow during topical application of different concentrations of bile acids to canine gastric mucosal surface. (Modified from Ritchie, 1983.)

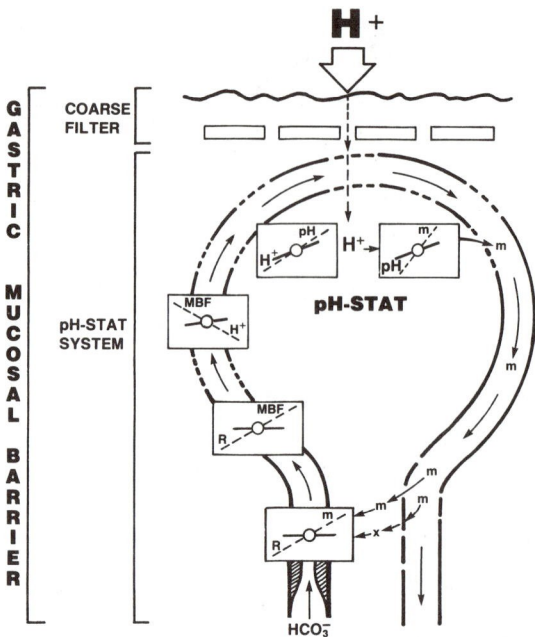

Figure 9. pH-stat model of the gastric mucosal barrier. The barrier is postulated to consist of a coarse filter (mucus + epithelial cell layer) and a blood flow-based pH-stat system. An increase in the interstitial hydrogen ion concentration is hypothesized to cause a mucosal pH-stat to release more vasoactive mediator(s) (m), which directly or indirectly (x), causes a decrease in submucosal arteriolar resistance (R). The resulting increase in local mucosal blood flow (MBF) restores the superficial interstitial pH to its normal value. The portions of the superficial mucosal vascular circuit drawn with short dashed lines represent capillary fenestrations. Mediator(s) (m) are hypothesized to be capable of causing increased permeability in basal venous vessels (long dashed lines) and/or of triggering a transendothelial increase of an arteriolar vasodilatory substance (x).

have not been defined. Neither the postulated pH-stat itself nor the regulatory mediator(s) has been clearly identified as such. However, a strong possible candidate for the pH-stat itself is the mucosal mast cell, and a good candidate for a primary mediator is histamine (see Section 4.4.2). Prostaglandins may also play an important role in this system. Clearly, more experimental work needs to be done in this area.

4.4. Mucosal Mast Cells

4.4.1. Mucosal Mast Cells in Pathophysiological Barrier Function

Thus far, mucosal barrier function has been described in terms of mechanisms to prevent superficial tissue damage. What happens when these defensive mechanisms begin to fail? Not surprisingly, additional barrier features assume prominence. One of the most striking is the blood flow response triggered by the mucosal mast cells (Fig. 10).

If mucosal defense is clearly failing, i.e., surface mucosal cells find themselves in an overwhelmingly hostile chemical environment, then superficial mucosal mast cells concertedly degranulate, releasing salvos of vasoactive mediators that trigger marked changes in mucosal blood flow. Venoconstriction and venospasm severely restrict venous drainage, while arterial blood flow into the same local area greatly increases. A plasma-filled blister is rapidly created at the site of mucosal injury. Under such conditions, blood flow not only delivers bicarbonate, oxygen, and nutrients, but it quickly and forcefully delivers plasma to dilute, push back, and retard further entry of offending chemicals, be they protons or xenobiotics. This effect is rather like the classic military defensive strategy of blowing up the bridges just in front of an advancing hostile army (venoconstriction) while simultaneously dynamiting an upstream dam (arterial dilation)—a defense reserved for desperate situations, but usually an effective one. This mucosal mast cell-mediated response most often suffices to limit necrotic damage to the relatively low-pressure capillary bed of the mucosa, preventing the more serious consequences of damage to the deeper higher-pressure submucosal arterial vessels. This response is described in more detail in Section 5.2.1. It is mentioned here to illustrate the key role that mucosal mast cells and mucosal blood flow play as part of gastric mucosal barrier function under some pathophysiological conditions.

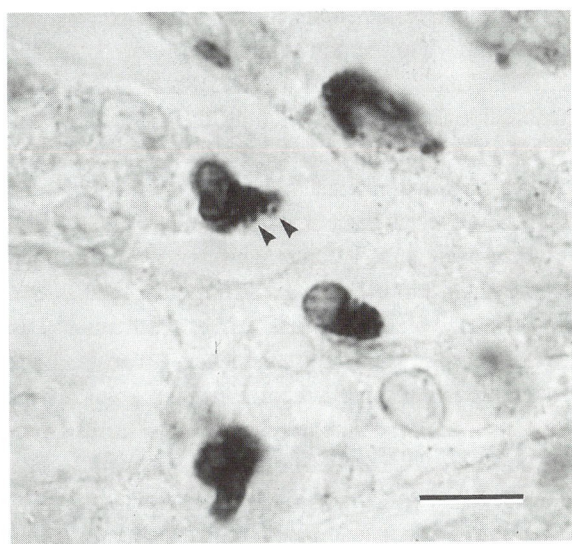

Figure 10. Cluster of typical metachromatically stained mucosal mast cells in the superficial gastric mucosa of the rat. Individual histamine-containing cytoplasmic granules can often be clearly discerned (e.g., arrowheads). Lead acetate fixation, toluidine blue staining with methyl orange counterstain. Bar = 20 μm.

4.4.2. Mucosal Mast Cells in Physiological Barrier Function?

Stationed in interstitial tissue in the upper third of the mucosa, mucosal mast cells appear to function as sentinels that monitor, and possible routinely fine-tune, the adequacy of local mucosal defense (Figs. 6 and 10). Their functional independence and widespread superficial distribution would permit monitoring and regulating mucosal defense in a highly localized way. Consistent with such a role, these cells, also called atypical mast cells, are notoriously sensitive to environmental perturbations, even more so than the familiar submucosal or typical mast cells. For example, most cells, including submucosal mast cells, can be preserved histologically with formalin. However, mucosal mast cells cannot. They discharge their inflammatory-mediator-laden granules in response to formalin and many other chemical fixatives. Thus these cells are unusually sensitive to environmental perturbation, which they respond to by releasing vasoactive chemicals that tend to restore local homeostasis. That is, they release mediators such as histamine that stimulate local bicarbonate production by parietal cells and promote plasma exudation into irritated sites. Histamine also enhances venular permeability, which fosters venous–arterial communication, and histamine directly causes arteriolar dilation. Thus, it can be suggested that the mucosal mast cell is an excellent candidate for the postulated mucosal pH-stat and that histamine constitutes a strong candidate as one of the mediators of the pH-stat system (Fig. 9). This would also be consistent with the observations made a decade ago by Bruggeman *et al.* (1979) that the luminal acid-dependent vasodilation that occurs in perfused canine gastric tissue is largely attributable to endogenously released histamine.

Contrary to the now classic view that mast cells and histamine are mucosal elements that contribute to ulceration, the view proposed here suggests that mucosal mast cells and histamine are elements that protect against ulceration. It is clear that, as emphasized in the classic view, intramucosally released histamine might stimulate acid secretion by parietal cells. However, it seems likely that the effect of histamine to stimulate local bicarbonate secretion from those same parietal cells, together with its effect to stimulate local blood flow, will be significantly more beneficial than detrimental to the local tissue. For the most part, protons secreted by parietal cells still have to find their way up through the gastric pits and back across the mucosal barrier. Even though the barrier may be leaky, elevating superficial proton influx, typically barrier function is still partly intact and will continue to reduce proton influx by several orders of magnitude. By contrast, virtually any and all bicarbonate secreted by the parietal cells will essentially be quantitatively and immediately available for transport up to the zone of superficial acidification, provided the situation has not gotten too far out of hand. As long as mucosal blood flow is intact, a leaky gastric mucosal barrier can be handled quite well by the mucosa (see Fig. 8). Moreover, luminal acid is necessary, but not sufficient, for lesion formation (see Section 5.1). Thus it is suggested that the determining element in the pathogenesis of acid-dependent mucosal lesions is the adequacy of the response of the mucosal pH-stat system. It is further hypothesized that the mucosal mast cell is a good candidate for the pH-stat itself and that histamine maybe an important mediator of the pH-stat system.

5. BLOOD FLOW IN MUCOSAL PATHOPHYSIOLOGY

In a number of circumstances, failure of the interlocking defenses of the gastric wall results in the formation of mucosal lesions. Clinically, the consequences can be serious. Until very recently, severe gastric bleeding was associated with a high mortality rate. Although bleeding from a chronic gastric ulcer is not uncommon, most cases of severe gastric bleeding are classified as stress ulcers. These acute mucosal lesions are associated with a variety of common clinical states of circulatory shock, viz. severe hemorrhage, trauma, sepsis, or cardiac failure. Some investigators also classify as stress ulcers the gastric lesions that follow central nervous system (CNS) trauma (Cushing's ulcers) or extensive body surface burns (Curling's ulcers). Gastric lesions quite similar to stress ulcers are also associated with the ingestion of certain types of drugs, notably nonsteroidal anti-inflammatory drugs (NSAID). An additional type of clinically common gastric lesion is acute topical gastritis, caused by mucosal contact with strongly concentrated substances from several chemical classes, e.g., alcohols, acids, bases, or salts.

This section applies the concepts discussed earlier in this chapter to specific examples from each of the above classes of clinically relevant lesions. The lesions are classified into two general categories: acid-dependent and acid-independent. Although most of the experimental studies cited below employed non-human mammalian tissue, there are no data to suggest any important species differences in lesion pathogeneses. It will be seen that in all cases in which the pathogenesis appears reasonably well understood, alteration of mucosal blood flow plays a fundamental role in lesion formation.

5.1. Acid-Dependent Lesions and Blood Flow

Acid-dependent mucosal lesions result from cell necrosis caused by cellular acidification. The ability of cells to maintain their intracellular pH depends on a number of factors, perhaps the most fundamental of which is not having to deal with an overwhelmingly high extracellular hydrogen ion concentration (see Section 4.3.3). In other words, the interstitial pH must be maintained in a range reasonably close to that of cytoplasmic pH. Blood flow is a key factor determining the extracellular muscosal pH (see Fig. 7); mucosal blood flow depends on mucosal resistance to flow and systemic blood pressure. This section discusses two examples of mucosal blood flow insufficiency resulting from a change in either one or the other of these two variables. In the first example, hemorrhagic shock, inadequate mucosal blood flow results largely from subnormal systemic blood pressure, a consequence of hypovolemia. In the second example, the indomethacin-induced lesion, insufficient mucosal blood flow is caused mainly by a pharmacologically induced increase in mucosal resistance to blood flow. The resulting lesions in the two cases are histologically very similar. As for aspirin-induced lesions, although the main pharmacological action of aspirin is similar to that of indomethacin, mucosal lesions induced by oral aspirin are histologically quite distinct from those caused by indomethacin. Thus, aspirin affords a good example of the importance of very localized effects of drugs on mucosal blood flow and on mucosal tissue. Finally, the possible role of insufficient mucosal blood flow in the etiology of chronic gastric ulcer is commented on.

5.1.1. Hemorrhagic Shock

The stomach wall does not autoregulate its blood flow; i.e., flow falls as perfusion pressure falls (see Section 3.1). In experimental models, it has been found that if the blood pressure falls below about 40 mm Hg, mucosal blood flow falls to about 33% of normal. This degree of reduction compromises the ability of the mucosal pH-stat mechanism to regulate intramural pH (Fig. 11). During the first 30 min prior to bleeding, the intramural pH monitored at mid-thickness of the mucosa was essentially constant, even though the transepithelial hydrogen ion gradient was increased roughly one million times by instilling in the gastric lumen 150 mM HCl instead of a neutral buffer. Moreover, even when the barrier to HCl influx was broken with 10 mM bile salt (+ TCA), intramural pH did not fall prior to bleeding, presumably because of the compensatory increase in mucosal blood flow (see Fig. 8). This illustrates the mucosal pH-stat system in normal operation.

However, if arterial blood pressure is lowered to 30–40 mm Hg, intramural acidification occurs (Fig. 11). Not shown are data indicating that the rate of loss of acid from the lumen (acid backdiffusion) is unaffected by the shocked state; i.e., the permeability of the barrier to HCl is the same both before and during shock. As expected, if the barrier is rendered leaky with topical bile salt

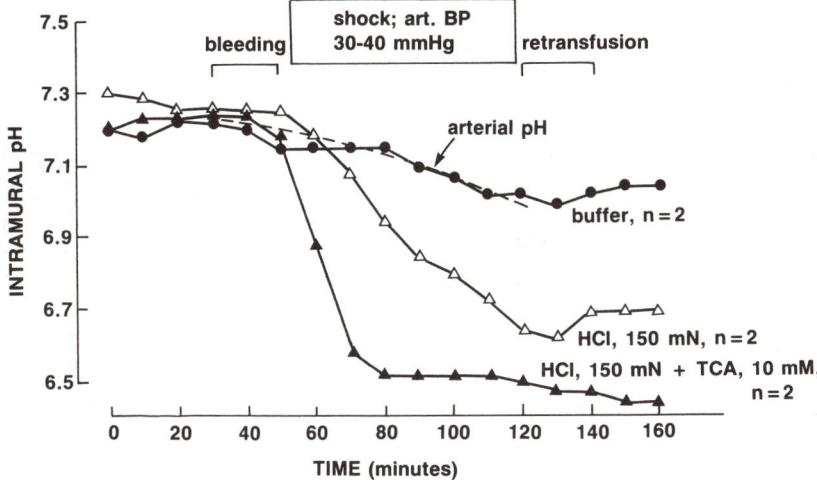

Figure 11. Intramural pH in canine stomach containing neutral buffer, 150 mN HCl or 150 mN HCl + 10 mM taurocholic acid (TCA) during hemorrhagic shock. (From Kivilaakso *et al.*, 1978.)

(+ TCA), intramural acidification occurs somewhat faster. Thus, in the shocked state, intramural acidification occurs, not because the barrier is broken, not because of the presence of bile salts, and not because basal blood flow is reduced per se, but because the very low systemic pressure renders the blood flow-dependent pH-stat mechanism ineffective.

The sequence of microscopic events leading to lesion formation in hemorrhagic shock is illustrated in Fig. 12. The normal honeycomb pattern of superficial mucosal flow (Fig. 12A) gradually fades as the blood pressure is lowered to roughly 35 mm Hg, while exposing the lumenal mucosal surface to 100 mM HCl (Fig. 12B). As mucosal blood flow fades, epicenters of acidification develop preferentially at the weakest points in the mucosal barrier, i.e., over capillary zones in the superficial vascular network (see Section 2.2.3; see also Fig. 3A). Any existing small mucosal defects will also serve as epicenters of acidification. Thus, centered primarily over the capillary zones of the superficial vascular network, hemispherical zones of superficial focal necrosis form because of the unopposed diffusion of acid into the bicarbonate- and blood flow-deprived mucosa.

Systemic acidosis associated with shock is a contributing, but not determining, factor of mucosal acidification. That is, in experimental models of hemorrhagic shock, even though systemic acidosis is prevented, lesions still form. Likewise, hypoxia contributes to lesion formation in two ways. First, lack of

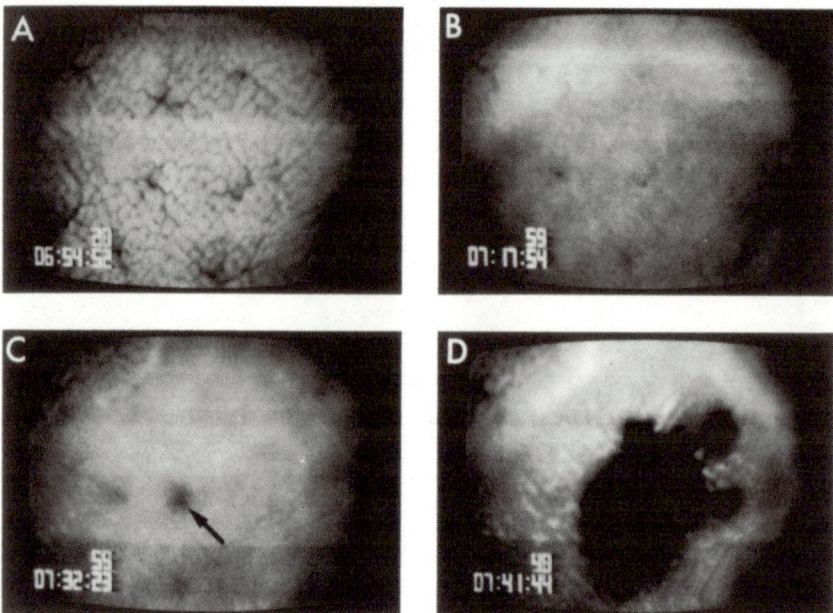

Figure 12. Photographs from a videomonitor of the luminal surface of the gastric mucosa of an anesthetized rat subjected to hemorrhagic shock. Magnification on the face of the videomonitor. (x120) (A) Control period with normotension and Kreb's solution applied to the luminal surface. A normal honeycomb-like superficial mucosal blood flow pattern is seen (cf. Fig. 3A). (B) Same scene at 27% of control blood pressure with 0.1 N HCl applied to the luminal surface during hypotension. The blood flow pattern has disappeared with only a slight trace of collecting venules remaining. (C) Same scene 7 min 31sec after retransfusion of blood. One bleeding point is seen (arrow). (D) Same scene approximately 17 min after retransfusion. More bleeding points are seen. (From Morishita and Guth, 1987.)

oxygen causes a general weakening of cellular resistance because of lowered cellular ATP levels. ATP is needed to power defensive secretions and protective ion pumps. Second, lack of oxygen from poor blood flow likely causes a buildup of organic acids from glycolytic metabolism. These would contribute to local tissue acidification. However, lesion development clearly depends on luminal acid. Therefore, tissue-derived acid must play only a minor contributory role in lesion formation. Likewise, mucosal ATP depletion does not appear to be pathogenetically critical, whereas mucosal acidification does, since erosions or bleeding do not occur in shocked tissue given supplemental intra-arterial bicarbonate under conditions that do not restore mucosal blood flow. Thus, in the hemorrhagic shock-induced lesion, superficial focal mucosal necrosis results primarily from luminal acid-dependent focal tissue acidosis that occurs because of the inability of the blood flow-dependent pH-stat mechanism to function properly.

When blood pressure is restored, blood re-enters the damaged tissue zone, resulting in hemorrhage (Fig. 12C,D). Bleeding usually occurs from the base of seemingly cone-shaped necrotic zones centered between collecting venules, i.e., centered over the superficial capillary zones (Fig. 13). Bleeding would be expected to initiate from the deepest portion of the lesion, since the microvascular capillary pressure will be slightly higher at the afferent than at the efferent end of a mucosal capillary. The zone of necrosis is presumably actually hemispherical rather than cone-shaped, hemispherical being the shape expected if luminal acid diffuses into the tissue from a weak point on the luminal surface. However, the hemodynamic forces that accompany bleeding from the basal aspect of the necrotic zone appear to cause red blood cells (RBC) and debris from the necrotic tissue to percolate up through the necrotic zone in a fanlike manner, contributing to the cone-shaped appearance of the final lesion (Fig. 13). Points of bleeding always occur from necrotic tissue zones, but not all necrotic zones bleed. This is most likely a question of the magnitude of local capillary pressure required to dislodge coagulated blood and tissue versus the magnitude of capillary pressure locally available to do so. This will vary from lesion to lesion, depending on local factors. In some cases, flow is momentarily restored before weakened capillaries burst. This probably results from additional damage brought on by the increase in capillary pressure accompanying reperfusion, as well as by the generation of tissue-damaging oxygen-derived free radicals that accompanies reperfusion in many tissues.

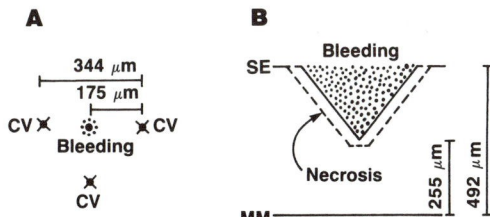

Figure 13. Schematic drawings of bleeding from the luminal gastric mucosal surface of rats subjected to hemorrhagic shock. (A) En face view. Bleeding occurs at points midway between collecting venules (CV) (cf. Fig. 3A). (B) Cross-sectional view. Bleeding occurs from the bottom of a conical zone of tissue necrosis in the outer half of the mucosa. SE, surface epithelium; MM, muscularis mucosae. (From Morishita and Guth, 1987.)

5.1.2. Indomethacin

Besides being a direct function of mean arterial pressure, mucosal blood flow is inversely dependent on mucosal resistance to flow (see Figs. 5 and 7). Thus, a state of high mucosal resistance to flow can result in a low-flow state that, in the presence of luminal acid, can give rise to mucosal lesions. This type of case is well illustrated by indomethacin, one of the best-studied cyclo-oxygenase inhibitors.

In general, the gastric lesions resulting from indomethacin are quite similar to those produced by hemorrhagic shock. The lesions are acid dependent and are preceded by mucosal blanching. A cross section through a typical indomethacin-induced mucosal lesion is shown in Fig. 14A. A cone-shaped zone of necrosis is seen to extend about halfway through the mucosa. Note the resemblance to the hemorrhagic shock-induced lesion (Fig. 13B). The lesion depicted in Fig. 14A resulted from intraperitoneal administration of indomethacin. A typical lesion resulting from oral administration of the drug is shown in Fig. 14B. The oral lesion is not distinguishable from the intraperitoneal lesion. Moreover, the frequency and the severity of such lesions are the same by either route of administration. Thus, the lesions result from a systemic, not a local, effect of indomethacin.

Indomethacin, especially at high doses, has a number of well-defined systemic effects. It causes constriction of arterioles in various tissues, thereby raising total peripheral resistance. Since it has no effect on cardiac output, indomethacin can slightly elevate mean arterial blood pressure (MAP) (Fig. 15). Despite this increase in MAP, a substantial reduction in gastric blood flow

Figure 14. Gastric mucosal lesions induced in rats by indomethacin, a nonsteroidal anti-inflammatory drug. (A) Indomethacin (100 mg/kg) was administered intraperitoneally and lesion formation was assessed 4 hr later. Note the resemblance to Fig. 13B. Labels as in Fig. 13B. (H & E stain.) Bar = 100 μm. (B) Conditions were the same as in Fig. 14A, except that indomethacin was administered per os. The lesion from the orally-administered drug is not distinguishable from that of the systemically administered drug (Fig. 14A), indicating the systemic rather than the topical nature of lesion formation with this drug. Labels as in Fig. 13B. (H & E stain.) Bar = 200μm.

Figure 17. Gastric lesion induced in rat mucosa by particulate aspirin (300 mg/kg) given per os. Note the distinctive appearance of this lesion compared with that shown for indomethacin in Fig. 14. A direct topical cytotoxic effect of particulate aspirin is suggested. (H & E stain.) Bar = 100μm.

Figure 18. Gastric lesion induced in rat mucosa by topical ethanol. Principal features are superficial contact necrosis with marked hyperemia and massive local edema. The semicircular cross-sectional profile of the lesion is indicative of blister formation. Fixation was done 30 min after ethanol administration. (H & E stain.) Bar = 200μm.

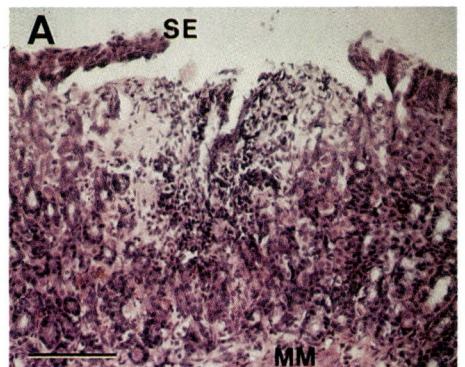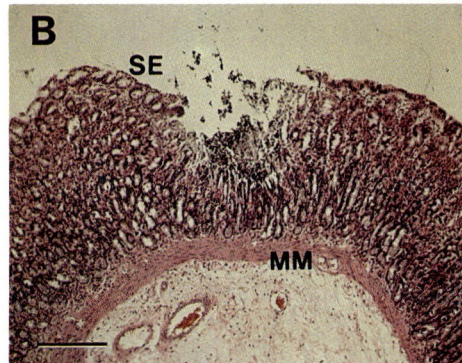

Figure 14

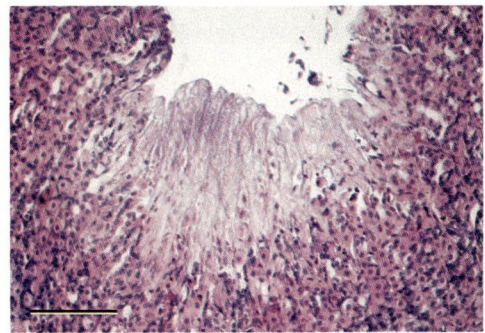

Figure 17

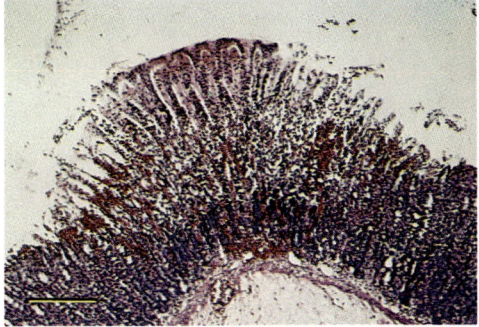

Figure 18

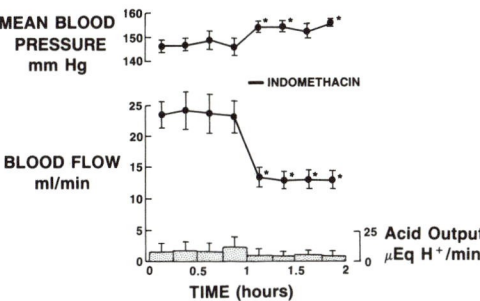

Figure 15. Changes in mean blood pressure, basal left gastric arterial flow, and gastric acid output produced by indomethacin (8 mg/kg, i.v.) in anesthetized dogs. Bars represent SEM. Asterisks (*) indicate $p < 0.05$ versus appropriate controls. (From Gerkens et al., 1977.)

occurs. Therefore, by definition, indomethacin causes an increased resistance to blood flow in gastric tissue:

$$\text{Resistance} = \text{pressure difference}/\text{blood flow}$$

Indomethacin appears to elevate resistance to gastric blood flow by two main effects. First, indomethacin causes constriction of gastric submucosal arterioles. Besides numerous flow measurements indicating this indirectly, videomicroscopic studies have directly shown that indomethacin causes constriction of gastric arterioles. This effect is probably linked to cyclo-oxygenase inhibition. However, whether it results primarily from a prostaglandin deficiency or from a direct or indirect active vasoconstrictive effect remains unclear. Since indomethacin is such a widely used experimental tool, this is an important point to clarify. The degree of reduction in basal blood flow by indomethacin is usually reported to be only about 50% (Fig. 15), which, by itself, may not be quite sufficient to precipitate significant lesion formation is an otherwise healthy mucosa. Indomethacin does not significantly enhance basal acid secretion (Fig. 15, bottom). Nor does systemic indomethacin increase the permeability of the mucosal barrier to acid.

A second way in which indomethacin can cause increased resistance to gastric blood flow is by its stimulatory effect on gastric muscular contractions. Such an effect on gastrointestinal (GI) motility may be related to the high degree of nonulcerative GI intolerance common to this class of drugs. Especially at hypertherapeutic doses, indomethacin induces a high-frequency, high-amplitude pattern of gastric contractions. In indomethacin-treated rats, a very strong correlation has been shown between drug-induced enhancement of gastric motility and the development of a mucosal lesion. Although cause and effect have not been clearly separated, it seems likely that gastric hypermotility might cause physical compression of one zone of the mucosal surface against another, resulting in blanching of superficial mucosal capillaries, such as occurs when the tips of two fingers are pressed together. Coupled with reduced mucosal capillary flow and pressure from indomethacin-induced arteriolar constriction, the ischemic mucosa would then be especially vulnerable to superficial acidification.

An important consequence of the indomethacin-induced increased resistance to flow is that the function of the mucosal pH-stat system is disrupted (Fig. 16). Indomethacin caused a significant depression of mucosal blood flow (MBF), either in the absence (ACID + INDO versus ACID) or in the presence of taurocholate (ACID + TAURO + INDO versus ACID + TAURO) (Fig. 16C). In neither case did indomethacin cause an increase in acid loss from the lumen (Fig. 16B). Thus, systemic indomethacin did not detectably enhance the permeability of the barrier to hydrochloric acid. It is also shown that (1) inclusion of surface-active taurocholate increased acid loss from the lumen by a factor of 3 (ACID versus ACID + TAURO) (Fig. 16B); (2) this was matched by a threefold increase in mucosal blood flow (Fig. 16C); and (3) no or very few erosions formed (Fig. 16A). However, when the protective mucosal blood flow response was blunted by indomethacin (ACID + TAURO + INDO versus ACID +

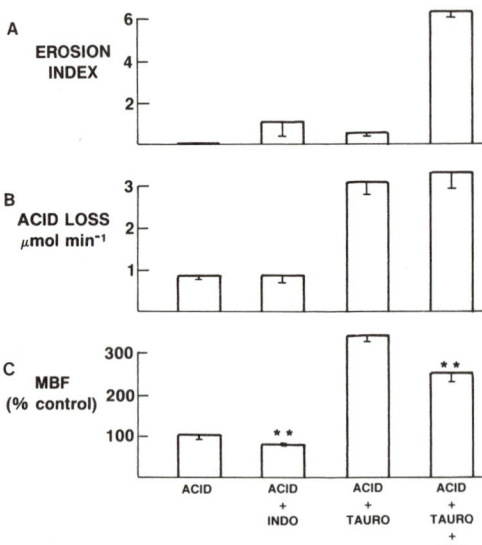

Figure 16. Effect of 3-hr gastric perfusion with the combinations (A,B,C) shown of 100 mN HCl (ACID), 2 mM taurocholate (TAURO), and 20 mg/kg, s.c., indomethacin (INDO) on mucosal erosion formation, acid backdiffusion, and mucosal blood flow (MBF) in the rat. Results are mean ±SEM. Asterisks indicate $p < 0.01$ versus appropriate controls. (From Whittle, 1980.)

TAURO) (Fig. 16C), a greatly elevated number of mucosal erosions resulted (ACID + TAURO + INDO versus ACID + TAURO) (Fig. 16A). Thus, although the pathogenetic particulars differ in some respects between indomethacin- and hemorrhagic shock-induced lesions, the two cases appear to share the same fundamental defensive defect, viz. the inability of the blood flow-dependent pH-stat mechanism to respond adequately to interstitial acidification.

5.1.3. Aspirin

Aspirin is a cyclo-oxygenase inhibitor, roughly 10 times less potent than indomethacin. Administered systemically, aspirin is capable of producing all the effects described above for indomethacin: slightly raised MAP, decreased gastric blood flow, mucosal blanching, and formation of mucosal lesions. Although clear data are unavailable, mucosal lesions produced by systemic aspirin presumably are indistinguishable from those described for indomethacin.

Aspirin is not usually taken parenterally, however, but most often is ingested orally in tablet form or as a suspension of particles. As was shown 50 years ago, contact of the gastric mucosa with aspirin particles elicits a strong, highly localized hyperemic response around each particle. The fact that the mucosa can respond in such a highly focal way should be kept in mind when gross measurements of mucosal blood flow are interpreted. This hyperemic response to aspirin particles is a defensive blood flow reaction that limits the pronounced local toxicity of concentrated aspirin. The local corrosive effect of particulate aspirin results in gastric lesions quite distinct from those caused by systemic cyclo-oxygenase inhibition (Fig. 17). For example, whereas many cellular nuclei are apparent in the indomethacin lesions shown in Fig. 14, virtually complete dissolution of nuclear structure occurs with topical aspirin (Fig. 17). Also, topical particulate aspirin is associated with histologically distinct craters in the mucosa, focal erosions where mucosal tissue appears to have literally been burned away.

Salicylate is a breakdown product of aspirin (acetylsalicylate). Salicylate is also a cyclo-oxygenase inhibitor, but a very weak one, some 1000 times less active than indomethacin. Given systemically, it does not cause gastric lesions, even at very high doses. However, given orally, particulate salicylate produces the same sort of local hyperemic response that aspirin does and also causes similar mucosal lesions. Importantly, environmental acid is necessary for salicylates to penetrate mucosal cell membranes and to cause cytotoxicity. Cytotoxicity from acidified salicylates results from a variety of direct toxic effects that are beyond the scope of this discussion. Suffice it to remember that in the presence of acid, salicylates have a pronounced local corrosive effect. This point is nicely illustrated by the well-known use of topical acidified salicylate preparations to dissolve warts.

5.1.4. Gastric Ulcer

More than 130 years ago, Virchow stated quite simply that gastric ulcer is caused by vascular insufficiency. This proposal has since been repeatedly advanced. However, very little can be said about the role of mucosal blood flow in chronic gastric ulcer. This is because relatively little is known about the etiology of chronic gastric ulcer and because there are no well-studied experimental animal models of this condition. Nevertheless, it can be said that extant information is consistent with an important role of deficient mucosal blood flow in chronic ulceration. For example, most gastric ulcer patients secrete normal or subnormal, not supernormal, amounts of hydrochloric acid. This has been interpreted by many to indicate that the underlying factor in gastric ulcers is a deficiency in mucosal defense, possibly in mucosal blood flow. Consistent with this notion, the strong anatomical proclivity of gastric ulcers to occur in the smaller curvature of the stomach has been argued by some to result from a relatively spare and vulnerable vascular network at that site. However, considerably more work in this area is needed before meaningful clear conclusions can be drawn regarding the role of mucosal blood flow in the pathogenesis of chronic gastric ulcer.

5.2. Acid-Independent Mucosal Lesions

A second major class of gastric lesions are those that are independent of luminal acid and in which mucosal blood inflow is supernormal rather than subnormal. These are the lesions of acute topical gastritis, typically caused by contact of the mucosa with strong chemical entities, such as concentrated acids, bases, alcohols, and salts. Gastric lesions caused by hot liquids probably also fall into this class. The best studied lesion of the topical necrotic type is that produced by concentrated ethanol. This is discussed first, followed by a few comments on other topical necrotizing agents.

5.2.1. Ethanol

The role of mucosal blood flow in the pathogenesis of acid-independent lesions is quite different from that discussed above for acid-dependent lesions.

Indeed, it can be said that if the acid-dependent lesions of shock and systemic cyclo-oxygenase inhibition result from too little blood inflow, the grossly visible part of acid-independent lesions results from too much blood inflow. A sense of this can be obtained from examining the distinctive histology of the ethanol-induced lesion, an example of which is shown at relatively low magnification in Fig. 18. Note that the mucosa appears to have literally exploded from within. In addition to topical contact necrosis, mucosal edema and congestive hyperemia are very marked. It is hoped that comparison of Fig. 18 with the histological features of acid-dependent lesions (e.g., Figs. 13B, 14, and 17) will convince the reader that the ethanol-induced lesion is of a quite different nature.

Whereas acid-dependent lesions often take an hour or more to become grossly visible, ethanol-induced lesions develop within minutes. Local mucosal protective mechanisms suddenly become rather overwhelmed with a high concentration of this barrier-penetrating cytotoxin. Concentrated alcohol, sometimes used as a histologic fixative, essentially fixes the superficial cells by dehydrating them, extracting membrane lipids, and precipitating cellular proteins (Fig. 18, top center). What follows is essentially the rapid formation of a hyperemic blister at the site of contact with concentrated alcohol. Blister formation results from pronounced microvascular changes that begin within seconds after ethanol is applied. Rapid and strong constriction of mucosal venules and veins inhibits further entry of ethanol into the system (Fig. 19). Venoconstriction is accompanied by rapid and vigorous arteriolar and arterial dilation. This combination of microvascular events causes marked engorgement of mucosal capillaries and greatly elevated capillary pressure. In conjunction with the permeability-enhancing effects of ethanol and tissue-derived inflammatory mediators, the high capillary pressure causes intense mucosal edema. The subepithelial interstitial pressure and volume rise high enough to blister the epithelium (see Fig. 18).

The blister-forming reaction of acute topical gastritis is thus essentially an acute inflammatory response. One important source of inflammatory mediators is the mucosal mast cell (see Fig. 10). Within 30 sec of exposure to concentrated ethanol, one half the superficial mast cells of rat gastric mucosal tissue discharge their histamine-containing intracellular granules. In addition to increasing venular permeability and possibly contributing to venoconstriction, histamine is capable of causing vigorous arteriolar dilation. Pharmacological studies have shown that ethanol-induced hyperemia depends on histamine acting at H_1-receptors, but not at H_2-receptors.

In addition to releasing histamine, stimulated mucosal mast cells are reported to synthesize and release a product of the lipoxygenase pathway, leukotriene C_4. Leukotriene C_4 has been shown to be a potent constrictor of gastric

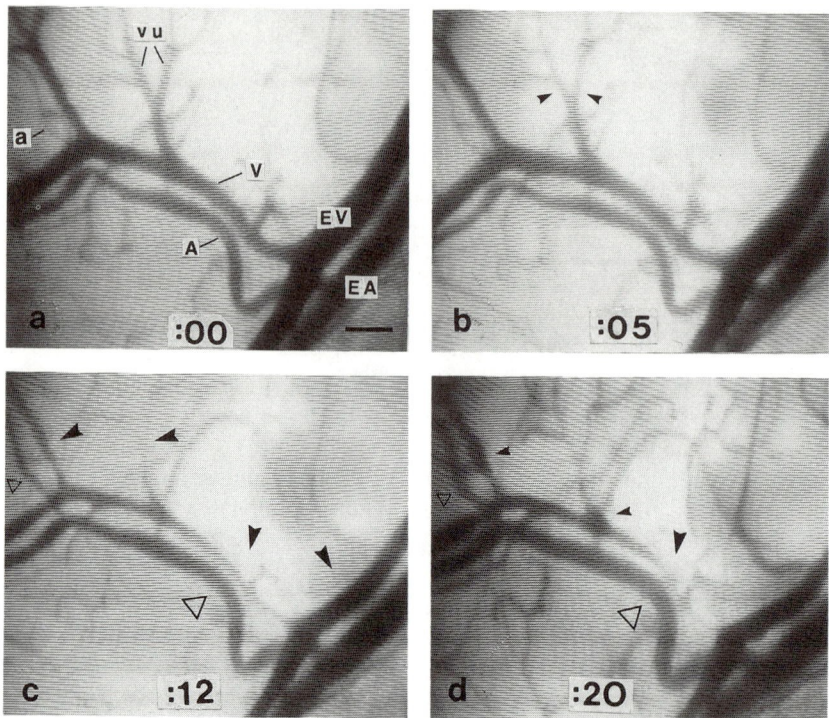

Figure 19. Frames from a low-magnification videotape recording showing a typical sequence of vascular events following intragastric infusion of ethanol in a rat stomach. The time in seconds after the midpoint of the 6-sec ethanol infusion is shown in the lower center of each picture. (a) Portion of the gastric vasculature after intraluminal saline infusion, just before the beginning of the ethanol infusion. Bottom right corner shows an external gastric artery (EA) giving rise to a small artery (A), which, having pierced the external muscle coat, sends a supplying arteriole (a) to the submucosal arteriolar plexus. Two venular branches (vu) that drain the deep mucosal venous plexus feed into a submucosal vein (V), which passes back up through the external muscle coat and empties into an external vein (EV). (b) The same field 5 sec after the intraluminal infusion of ethanol. The smaller venular segments closer to the mucosa are in the process of constricting (e.g., arrowheads). The larger vessels show little or no change. (c) The same field 12 sec after ethanol administration. Virtually all the postcapillary vessels present have constricted (e.g., black arrowheads). By contrast, the submucosal supplying arteriole (a) has dilated markedly (small clear arrowhead), and an increase in the diameter of artery (A) is detectable (large clear arrowhead). (d) The same area 20 sec after ethanol administration. Intense constriction persists in the submucosal vein (e.g., large dark arrowhead), while arteriole (a) and artery (A) have dilated markedly (small and large clear arrowheads, respectively). Note the focal areas of venular engorgement (small dark arrowheads). Bar = 500 μm. (From Oates and Hakkinen, 1988.)

venules and to be generated by the mucosa in response to contact with ethanol. Moreover, pharmacological studies indicate that in addition to being mediated by histamine, ethanol-induced hyperemic blister formation is also dependent on activity of the lipoxygenase pathway (Table II). Indomethacin, a cyclo-oxygenase inhibitor, had no effect on the percentage of mucosal corpus surface area that was hyperemic following ethanol challenge. By contrast, BW755C and nordihydroguaiaretic acid (NDGA), two structurally distinct lipoxygenase–cyclo-oxygenase inhibitors, each strongly suppressed ethanol-induced hyperemia. Co-administration of indomethacin and BW755C before ethanol challenge (Table II, INDO + BW755C) caused the same effect as BW755C alone, suggesting that the effectiveness of BW755C results not from enhanced prostaglandin formation, but from blocking the formation of one or more products of the lipoxygenase pathway, probably leukotriene C_4.

These results, together with additional data including histological and microvascular findings (e.g., Figs. 18 and 19), are integrated in a model recently proposed for the pathogenesis of the ethanol-induced lesion (Fig. 20). Further research is needed to clarify the identities and actions of the mediators that trigger the microvascular changes induced by topical ethanol.

The apparent purpose of the acute inflammatory response to topical concentrated ethanol is to dilute and prevent further entry of this cytotoxic substance into mucosal tissue (see Section 4.4.1). Damage is thus mostly confined to the relatively low-pressure rapidly healing superficial mucosa, while the regenerative zone deeper in the tissue and the higher-pressure submucosal arterioles and small arteries are protected to the extent possible. A topic of keen current interest is the cytoprotective effect of prostaglandins. This refers to the effect of prostaglandins on mucosal tissue to somehow prevent the ethanol-induced acute

Table II. Dependence of Ethanol-Induced Gastric Hyperemia on Activity of the Lipoxygenase Pathway[a]

Test substance	Dose (p.o.; mg/kg)	% Hyperemia	
		$\bar{x}$ ±SEM	N
Vehicle	—	17.4 ± 1.7	30
Indomethacin	20	14.8 ± 2.7	15
BW755C	10	6.2 ± 1.8	15[b]
BW755C	100	3.2 ± 1.0	15[b]
NDGA	100	2.9 ± 0.7	15[b]
INDO + BW755C	20 + 10	4.4 ± 0.9	15[b,c]

[a]From Oates and Hakkinen (1988).
[b]$p < 0.01$ versus vehicle control (Student's t-test).
[c]$p > 0.30$ versus BW755C at 10- (or 100-) mg/kg (Student's t-test).

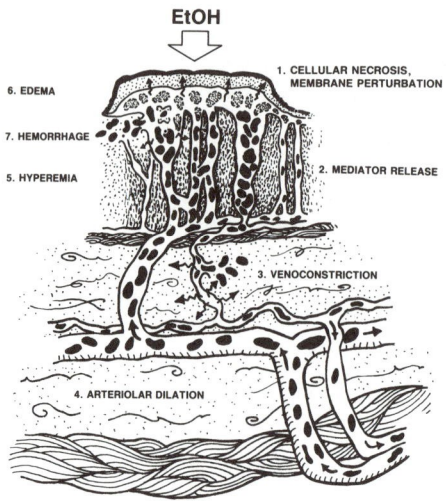

Figure 20. Proposed model for the pathogenesis of ethanol-induced gastric damage. Concentrated ethanol contacts the superficial gastric epithelium, causing necrosis and perturbation of superficial epithelial, endothelial, and mucosal mast cells (1), resulting in vasoactive mediator release (2), which triggers venoconstriction (3) and plasma exudation (wiggly arrows). Dilation of arterioles and arteries rapidly follows (4), leading to marked congestive hyperemia (5), edema (6), and hemorrhage (7). Further penetration of concentrated ethanol into the congested tissue causes hemolysis in congested capillaries and generalized protein precipitation, resulting in total stasis of blood flow in the immediate area. (From Oates and Hakkinen, 1988.)

inflammatory response from developing. The mechanism of this effect is an intriguing question. If it were merely a direct suppression of the acute inflammatory response itself, it is surprising that the amount of histologically evident cell necrosis in cytoprotected mucosae is not greater. By contrast, if the inflammatory process does not occur because it is unnecessary when the mucosal cells are in the cytoprotected state, what is the nature of this state of remarkably increased mucosal resistance to cytotoxins? Perhaps both possibilities pertain in part. *In vitro* studies of mucosal cell resistance should help shed some light on this fundamental issue.

5.2.2. Other Topical Necrotizing Agents

On contact with the gastric mucosa, a variety of strongly concentrated chemicals produce lesions similar to those caused by ethanol. Examples include concentrated HCl, NaOH, NaCl, and other alcohols, such as methanol or propanol. Hot water also produces similar lesions. Clearly, the effect is a nonspecific one. In addition, the pharmacological responses of these lesions are similar to one another as well as to the ethanol lesion. It is therefore probable that the mechanism of lesion formation is a common one, that is, largely independent of the particular necrotizing agent used and primarily dependent on mucosal tissue-derived mediators released in response to nonspecific trauma. One likely source of such mediators is the mucosal mast cell, well known to degranulate in response to a variety of nonspecific irritants. It seems likely that the model proposed for the ethanol-induced lesion (Fig. 20) is applicable in principle to a variety of other topical necrotizing agents.

5.3. The Mucosal Homeostat System: A Unifying Hypothesis

5.3.1. Existence of a Mucosal Homeostat System

Evidence was presented that the mucosa monitors and maintains a constant intramural pH by means of a blood flow-linked pH-stat system (see Sections 4.3.3 and 5.1.1). The basic mucosal response to a decrease in superficial interstitial pH is to increase mucosal arterial inflow as needed to restore and maintain interstitial pH. By contrast, there is also evidence that (1) the mucosa also responds with a marked increase in arterial inflow to concentrated luminal ethanol, and (2) the essential characteristics of mucosal response to concentrated ethanol also occur with various other concentrated substances, such as NaOH (see Section 5.2). Keeping in mind that the lesions produced by concentrated ethanol, NaOH and the like are, by definition, not dependent on luminal acid, it is clear that, even though ethanol and these other substances are barrier breakers, the increased arterial inflow in mucosae exposed to these substances is not likely to depend on mucosal acidification. This is particularly true in the case of mucosae exposed to concentrated NaOH. These observations imply that, in addition to the proposed pH-stat system (see Section 4.3.3), the mucosa has within it a mechanism or a system for sensing and responding to nonspecific perturbations in local mucosal homeostasis. This system is referred to as the mucosal homeostat system.

5.3.2. Nature of the Mucosal Homeostat

Is the homeostat system the same system as the pH-stat system? Quite possibly, yes. Since pH regulation is postulated to be accomplished largely through increased mucosal blood flow (see Fig. 9), this system could also serve to restore any other type of local environmental perturbation, such as a change in osmolarity. That is, the nature of the pH regulatory response is such as to maintain total environmental homeostasis, not simply pH.

The question then becomes whether the homeostat is the same as the pH-stat. In principle, the function of detecting and responding to local environmental change could reside almost anywhere in the mucosa—in superficial epithelial cells, in blood or plasma components, in certain specialized cells, or in some combination of these. However, the mucosal mast cell presents itself as a virtually ideal candidate for the job (see Section 4.4.2). And, on the basis of current knowledge, it really has no close competitor. Scattered throughout the upper third of the mucosa, mucosal mast cells are certainly in the right location. While they may be considered to constitute a network of microscopic monitors implanted in the superficial mucosa, the independent nature of each unit allows for very localized regulatory control. Within the present context, their unusual sensitivity to a variety of nonspecific environmental perturbations is precisely the sensory equipment needed. In addition, they are well equipped for generating and releasing vasoactive mediators capable of influencing local homeostasis, such as histamine and leukotriene C_4. Moreover, since mucosal mast cells are located interstitially very close to the fenestrated capillary endothelial cells, they are well positioned for efficient vasoregulation. Thus, it is not unreasonable to propose that mucosal mast cells are likely to constitute the (or at least a) major element of the mucosal homeostat.

5.3.3. Functioning of the Homeostat System

Broadening the pH-stat concept (see Section 4.3.3) to a homeostat concept permits the emergence of a unified view of the role of mucosal blood flow in mucosal defense (Fig. 21). The gastric mucosal barrier can then be conceptualized as being composed of two elements: a largely structural coarse filter and a largely functional homeostat system. The coarse filter corresponds to the mucus-covered epithelium and functions to reduce logarithmically the concentration of hydrogen ions or other irritants such as ethanol that might seek to enter the mucosal interstitium. Hydrogen ions or ethanol molecules that do enter are then handled by the blood flow-based homeostat system. The homeostat, probably consisting largely of mucosal mast cells, monitors one or more indices of interstitial homeostasis (pH, osmolarity, . . . ?). Relatively mild excursions from accepted norms of homeostasis are responded to with dollops of vasodilatory mediator(s) (m), probably histamine in many circumstances. Prostaglandins may also play an important role in this system. Increased venous levels of vasodilatory mediators are hypothesized to cause local arteriolar dilation and increased capillary flow, restoring local homeostasis. Under conditions of mild irritation, injury occurs only if blood flow or bicarbonate delivery is compromised.

Under conditions of increasing severity of disturbance in local superficial homeostasis, a threshold will be reached at which the maximal mucosal blood flow by itself is unable to preserve local homeostasis. It is hypothesized that the homeostat responds to this situation by releasing a second type of vasoactive mediator, a venoconstrictor, probably leukotriene C_4 (L). The local venocon-

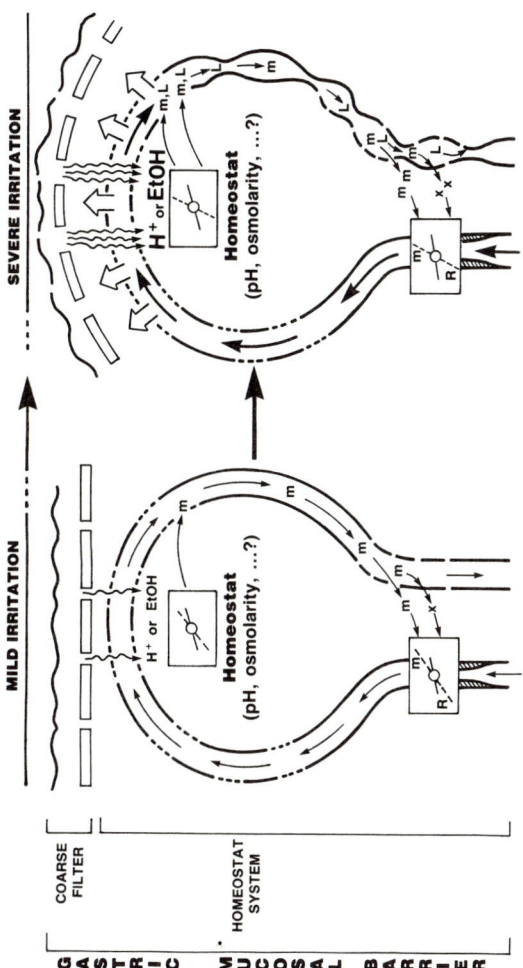

Figure 21. Homeostat model of the gastric mucosal barrier. The barrier is postulated to consist of a coarse filter (mucus and epithelial cells) and of a blood flow-based homeostat system. Mild perturbations of mucosal interstitial homeostasis are hypothesized to cause a mucosal homeostat to release an increased amount of one or more mediators (m), which directly or indirectly (x) causes a decrease in submucosal arteriolar resistance (R). This results in an increase in local mucosal blood flow that restores superficial mucosal homeostasis, preventing mucosal injury. Severe irritation is hypothesized to elicit the additional production of a venoconstrictive substance, (L), which synergizes with arterial vasodilatory substances (m), to restore local superficial homeostasis via local edema formation (large open arrows). EtOH, ethanol.

strictive effect of this second mediator synergistically enhances the superficial effect of increased arterial inflow to restore, or attempt to restore, local homeostasis by edema production. Under conditions of very severe irritation, hyperemic blister formation results.

Thus, it is hypothesized that under the control of the homeostat system, the mucosa is capable of mounting a full spectrum of protective blood flow responses to a potentially limitless variety of chemical insults. Depending on the severity of an insult, protective blood flow responses range from mild hyperemia to acute hemorrhagic blistering. In all cases, the aim is to restore local mucosal homeostasis.

6. SUMMARY AND CONCLUSIONS

Gastric mucosal blood flow plays a central role in preventing damage to the gastric lining. The remarkable effectiveness of this vascular defensive system is rooted in a profound integration of vascular structure and function with mucosal needs. This occurs at all levels of gastric tissue organization, from the gross arterial anastomotic network, to the unique upward flow design of the mucosal microvasculature, to the ultrastructure of mucosal capillaries and collecting venules.

The basic intramucosal defensive response is to increase arterial inflow to restore a disturbed extracellular environment. For example, when there is abnormally high permeability of the epithelial cell layer to HCl, mucosal flow increases in a linear fashion as a function of incoming protons. Mucosal blood flow thus appears to be an integral component of a mucosal system that maintains tissue homeostasis. This system is referred to as the mucosal homeostat system. Circulatory shock or pharmacologic inhibition of gastric cyclo-oxygenase can blunt the homeostat-mediated protective rise in mucosal blood flow. This makes the mucosa unusually vulnerable to even relatively small amounts of luminal acid and can result in mucosal erosions and hemorrhage. Better understanding of the pathogenesis of stress ulcers has led to significant improvements in clinical practice regarding the approach to the patient in circulatory shock. This includes aggressive prophylactic use of antacids and antisecretory agents, prevention of sepsis, volume replacement, treatment of cardiac abnormalities, and careful monitoring of systemic acid–base balance. Such measures have resulted in a drastic reduction in the incidence of severe gastric bleeding in shock patients in critical care units in recent years.

Clearly, aspirin, indomethacin, and other cyclo-oxygenase inhibitors should be used with great caution in patients with a prior history of upper GI bleeding and not at all in patients with active gastric or duodenal ulcer. Ingestion of this class of drugs with milk or meals to stimulate protective gastric blood flow is likely to reduce the incidence of mucosal bleeding. Concomitant antacids or antisecretory agents are sometimes also employed for this purpose.

Besides protecting mucosal tissue from infiltrating gastric acid, mucosal blood flow constitutes an important aspect of tissue resistance to nonspecific chemical assaults. If a high concentration of a noxious substance begins to damage superficial mucosal cells, the mucosa adds the tactic of venous constriction to the standard response of arteriolar dilation. Besides restricting further entry of the noxious substance into the portal circulation, venoconstriction synergizes with enhanced arterial inflow to flood the damaged superficial tissue zone forcefully with plasma, providing a very rapid and vigorous local countermeasure to the invading cytotoxic substance.

The available data suggest that this acute inflammatory response results from the release of histamine and leukotriene C_4, both possibly largely derived from mucosal mast cells. These cells are located superficially in the mucosa and are unusually sensitive to environmental perturbation. It is suggested that mucosal mast cells constitute a tissue homeostat, i.e., a tissue element responsible for monitoring and regulating intratissue environmental homeostasis. It is hypothesized that mucosal mast cells play an important role in maintaining the composition and pH of superficial interstitial fluid by responding to environmental perturbations with release of vasoactive mediators that modulate mucosal blood flow so as to maintain local mucosal homeostasis.

In the presence of cytoprotective agents, the mast cell-mediated inflammatory response to topical necrotic agents does not occur. Whether this is because the inflammatory reaction is no longer needed, i.e., the mucosal cells are protected by some other means, or because the inflammatory response itself is antagonized by cytoprotective agents, or both, is not yet clear. In this regard, *in vitro* studies of mechanisms by which mucosal cells develop enhanced resistance to environmental insults are of interest. The possible clinical benefits of cytoprotective substances are currently under study.

Finally, although considerable progress has been made in this area, much research remains to be done regarding the mechanisms by which mucosal blood flow participates in mucosal homeostasis. As these studies progress over the coming years, we can look forward to developing an even deeper appreciation of the critically important role played by gastric blood flow in mucosal defense.

ACKNOWLEDGMENTS. I am grateful for the support of Dr. Thomas Beyer and Dr. Nancy Hutson and for the excellent technical assistance of Pauline Gaudreau and John Hakkinen with the histology. The expert secretarial assistance of Doreen Gale is also gratefully acknowledged, as is additional help in this regard from Deborah Sanford, Kathryn Smith, and Daisy Johnson. Skillful assistance with the artwork from Bud Tucker, Gail Welch, Anita Parker, and Carol Milne is also greatly appreciated. Finally, a very large debt of gratitude is owed my wife, Nancy, for her continuous encouragement and patient support of this project.

ANNOTATED BIBLIOGRAPHY

Bruggeman TM, Wood JG, Davenport HW: Local control of blood flow in the dog's stomach: Vasodilation caused by acid back-diffusion following topical application of salicylic acid. *Gastroenterology* **77**:736–44, 1979.

> An important study on the mechanism of acid-induced mucosal vasodilation. It emphasizes the vasodilatory role of histamine when the mucosal barrier is broken with salicylic acid.

Cheung LY, Ashley SW: Gastric blood flow and mucosal defense mechanisms. *Clin Invest Med* **10**: 201–208, 1987.

> A good recent review covering techniques of mucosal blood flow measurement and emphasizing the importance of adequate mucosal blood flow in a clinical context.

Enerbäck L: Mast cells in rat gastrointestinal mucosa. *Acta Pathol Immunol Microbiol Scand [A]* **66**: 289–302, 1966.

> A classic paper describing the existence and unusual properties of gastrointestinal mucosal mast cells.

Gannon B, Browning J, O'Brien P, et al: Mucosal microvascular architecture of the fundus and body of human stomach. *Gastroenterology* **86**:866–75, 1984.

> Together with a 1982 companion study on the rat gastric microvasculature, some important morphological observations emphasizing anatomical aspects of local bicarbonate transport from parietal cells to superficial epithelial cells.

Gerkens JF, Shand DG, Flexner C, et al: Effect of Indomethacin and aspirin on gastric blood flow and acid secretion. *J. Pharmacol Exp Ther* **203**:646–652, 1977.

> A lucid study of the acute effects of systemic cyclo-oxygenase inhibition on key cardiovascular and gastric parameters.

Guth PH, Leung FW: Physiology of the gastric circulation, in Johnson LR (ed): *Physiology of the Gastrointestinal Tract,* ed. 2. New York, Raven Press, 1987, pp. 1031–1053.

> A comprehensive review of the gastric circulation and of experimental and clinical techniques for measuring gastric blood flow.

Holm-Rutili L, Öbrink KJ: Rat gastric mucosal microcirculation *in vivo. Am J. Physiol* **248**:G741– 746, 1985.

> An important study which quantitatively defines key structural and functional aspects of the superficial microvascular network in the rat gastric mucosa.

Kivilaakso E, Fromm D, Silen W: Relationship between ulceration and intramural pH of gastric mucosa during hemorrhagic shock. *Surgery* **84**:70–78, 1978.

One of the earliest and clearest demonstrations of the relationship between intramural acidification and lesion formation. This paper also highlights the critical importance of the capacity of the mucosa to dispose of influxing protons vis à vis the actual magnitude of influxing protons.

Morishita T, Guth PH: Effect of exogenous acid on the rat gastric mucosal microcirculation in hemorrhagic shock. *Gastroenterology* **92**:1958–64, 1987.

An insightful videomicroscopic and histological examination of the mechanism of lesion formation in experimental hemorrhagic shock. Of note is the observation that mucosal bleeding usually begins where superficial blood flow was lowest, i.e., at sites midway between mucosal collecting venules.

Oates PJ, Hakkinen JP: Studies on the mechanism of ethanol-induced gastric damage in rats. *Gastroenterology* **94**:10–21, 1988.

A recent study showing that gastric mucosal venoconstriction as well as arterial dilation occurs in response to a strong nonacid challenge such as concentrated ethanol. This study emphasizes the possible pathogenetic role of mucosal mast cell-derived histamine and leukotriene C_4 in ethanol-induced lesion formation.

Ritchie WP: Pathogenesis of acute gastric mucosal injury. *Viewpoints Dig Dis* **15**:17–20, 1983.

A succinct, readable article emphasizing the enhancement of mucosal blood flow as a critical mucosal protective mechanism and the importance of preventing mucosal acidosis.

Starlinger M, Jakesz R, Matthews JB, et al: The relative importance of HCO_3^- and blood flow in the protection of rat gastric mucosa during shock. *Gastroenterology* **81**:732–735, 1981.

One of the clearest *in vivo* demonstrations of the critical importance to the gastric mucosa of bicarbonate delivery via mucosal blood flow. Also notable is the *in vivo* demonstration that carbonic anhydrase activity appears to be necessary for mucosal bicarbonate to be effective.

Whittle BJR: Actions of prostaglandins on gastric mucosal blood flow, in Fielding LP (ed): *Gastrointestinal Mucosal Blood Flow*. Edinburgh, Churchill Livingstone, 1980, pp. 180–191.

A concise overview of prostaglandin, indomethacin, and taurocholate effects on the gastric mucosa. The important protective role of enhanced mucosal blood flow is pointed up.

Whittle BJR, Vane JR: Prostanoids as regulators of gastrointestinal function, in Johnson LR (ed): *Physiology of the Gastrointestinal Tract,* ed 2. New York, Raven Press, 1987, pp. 143–180.

A comprehensive review of the roles of prostanoids in gastrointestinal function, including important sections on the effects of prostanoids and nonsteroidal anti-inflammatory agents on gastric mucosal blood flow and on other components of the gastric barrier.

III

Cytoprotective Therapy

9

Cytoprotective Therapy
Prostaglandins

DONALD E. WILSON

1. INTRODUCTION

Prostaglandins are 20-carbon cyclic fatty acids synthesized from dietary fatty acids by virtually all mammalian cells. These naturally occurring compounds are biologically active, affect most cellular functions, and have both physiologic and pharmacologic effects in animals and in humans. Prostaglandins (PG) represent one of two known groups of arachidonic acid metabolites, collectively known as eicosanoids (Fig. 1). Because of their gastric acid antisecretory effects, as well as their ability to enhance gastroduodenal mucosal integrity, PG have undergone extensive evaluation in animals and in human subjects as potential antiulcer drugs. Naturally occurring PG are rapidly metabolized by enzyme systems present in most tissues, particularly in the lungs, liver, and gastrointestinal (GI) tract, so that their actions are short-lived, unless they are administered by constant infusion in relatively high concentrations. A number of metabolically stable PG analogues have been synthesized that are not only more potent than their natural counterparts but are also active by the oral route. This chapter reviews some of the data supporting a physiologic and therapeutic role for PG in maintaining mucosal integrity.

DONALD E. WILSON • Department of Medicine, State University of New York, Health Science Center at Brooklyn, Brooklyn, New York 11203.

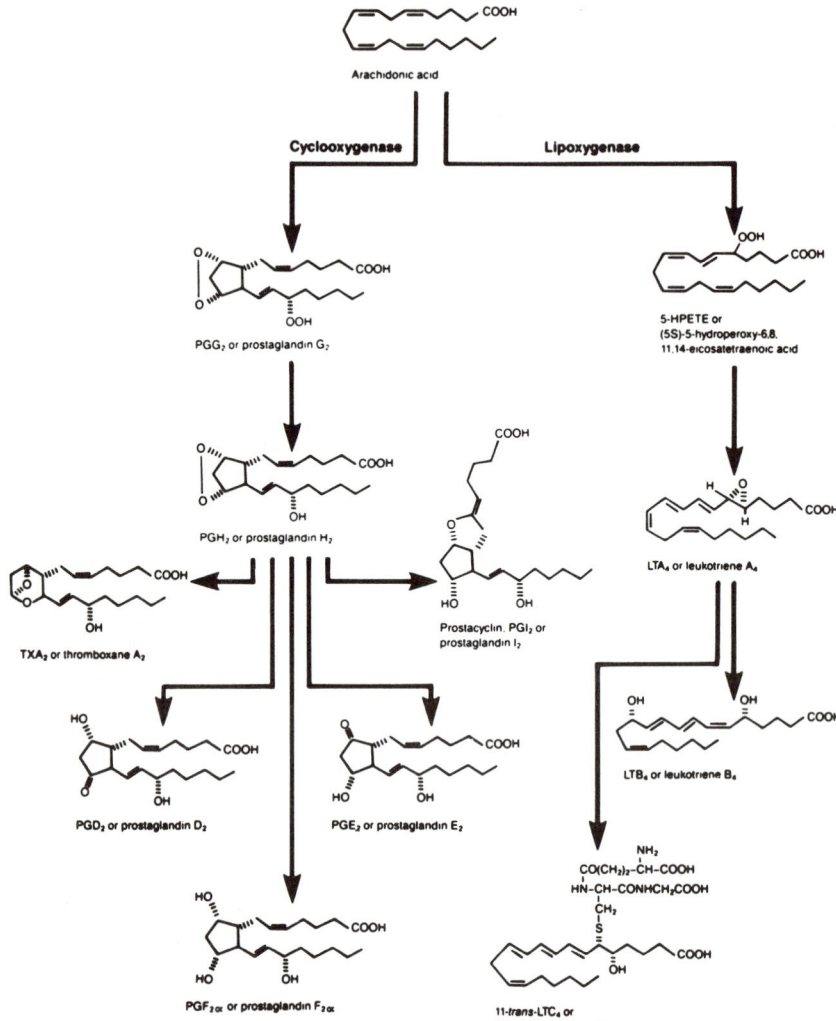

Figure 1. Biosynthesis of eicosanoids from arachidonic acid, detailing cyclo-oxygenase and lipoxygenase pathways.

2. EVIDENCE FOR A ROLE OF PROSTAGLANDIN IN CYTOPROTECTION

2.1. Experimental Models

2.1.1. Acid-Related Injury: Aspirin, NSAID, Bile Acids, Stress, Steroids, Secretagogues

André Robert and co-workers (1968) first reported that prostaglandin E_1 (PGE$_1$) could prevent pyloric ligation and corticosteroid-induced gastric ulceration in the rat. This observation, in and of itself, was not particularly surprising, since PGE$_1$ is a potent gastric acid antisecretory compound and since numerous reports in the literature indicated that the inhibition or neutralization of gastric acid could ameliorate the effects of stress and other types of experimental ulceration in animals. Several years later, in expanded and more detailed studies, Robert's group reported that several prostaglandins were capable of preventing or reducing gastric mucosal damage caused by indomethacin and flurbiprofen, nonsteroidal anti-inflammatory drugs (NSAID) that require the presence of acid to cause damage. In collaboration with Jacobson, Robert coined the term cytoprotection to describe this new phenomenon. Two important observations were made in this study: (1) nonantisecretory PG as well as antisecretory PG prevented gastric mucosal damage, and (2) antisecretory PG were protective at dosages well below (usually as little as 1/100) their effective antisecretory concentrations. It was also noted that when administered orally PG were three to five times as potent as when given subcutaneously and were also effective when given orally within 1 min of administration of the noxious agent, as compared with a 5-min pretreatment interval requirement following the subcutaneous route.

Both PGE$_2$, an antisecretory vasodilator, and PGF$_{2\alpha}$, a nonantisecretory vasoconstrictor, prevented the gastric damage, indicating that other common PG effects must be involved in the cytoprotective phenomenon. In later studies, Robert and other investigators (1971, 1979) were able to show that PG cytoprotection in the gastroduodenum was effective against a variety of acid-dependent noxious agents, including bile acids, hypertonic solutions, steroids, and secretagogues.

2.1.2. Non-Acid-Related Injury: Strong Acid or Alkali, Ethanol, Thermal Injury

Strong acids or bases such as 0.6 M HCl and 0.2 M NaOH, respectively, damage gastric mucosal cells by direct contact and, as such, do not require the presence of acid to cause necrosis. This is also true for 100% ethanol and thermal injury, such as that caused by the instillation of boiling water into the stomach. Robert *et al.* (1979) reported that PG could prevent damage caused by these acid-independent experimental ulcerogens in the rat. In these studies, PGE_2 and several PG analogues, 16,16-dimethyl PGE_2, 15(R)- and 15(S)-15 methyl $PGF_{2\beta}$, and 16,16-dimethyl PGA_2, prevented gastric necrosis by a variety of these noxious agents and did so in a dose-dependent manner, with the oral route more effective than subcutaneous administration.

The observations that antisecretory as well as nonantisecretory PG prevent gastric mucosal damage caused by both acid-dependent and acid-independent damaging agents, represented a milestone in our understanding of mucosal integrity and protection (Table I).

2.1.3. Direct and Adaptive Cytoprotection

In 1980, Robert's group made another important observation leading to increased understanding of the role of PG in mucosal protection. Using the rat, these workers observed that mild irritants, such as 0.15–0.35 M HCl, 5 mM acidified taurocholate, or 10–25% ethanol did not damage the gastric mucosa. Moreover, when a mild irritant was given orally to the animal 15 min prior to administering a strong irritant e.g., 80 mM taurocholate, the stomach was protected from the damage usually caused by the strong irritant. Robert further observed that when indomethacin was given to the animals before administration of the mild irritant, to prevent endogenous PG synthesis, subsequent protection against the damaging effects of the strong irritant did not occur. He reasoned that the mild irritants were stimulating endogenous PG synthesis in the gastric mucosa, accomplishing the subsequent protection against damage by the strong irritant. Having previously demonstrated exogenous mucosal protection by PG, Robert developed the concept of direct and adaptive cytoprotection (Fig. 2).

Several investigators have shown that Robert's hypothesis was indeed correct. Following the administration of a mild irritant such as 20% ethanol to a rat,

Table I. Causes of Gastric Mucosal Injury
Prevented by Prostaglandins

Ethanol
Aspirin, bile acids
Nonsteroidal anti-inflammatory drugs (NSAID)
Stress
Hypertonic/hypotonic solutions
Caustic solutions (lye, boiling water)

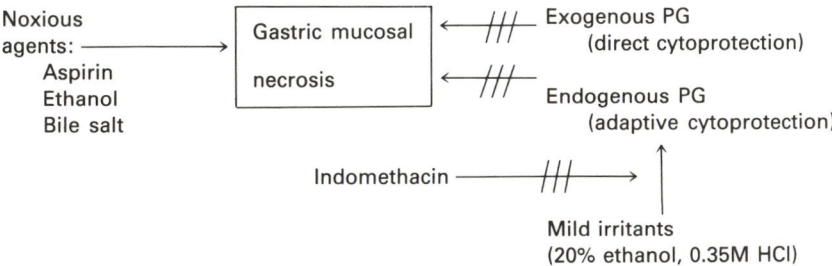

Figure 2. Diagrammatic representation of direct and adaptive cytoprotection by prostaglandins. Pretreatment with mild irritants induces adaptive cytoprotection, preventing damage caused by strong irritants. Adaptive cytoprotection is prevented by pretreatment with indomethacin.

one can measure a subsequent significant stimulation of mucosal synthesis of PGE_2, PGI_2, and $PGF_{2\alpha}$. The demonstration of direct and adaptive cytoprotection provides significant support for the concept that PG have a physiologic role in maintaining the normal integrity of the gastric mucosa.

2.2. Effects of Modifiers of Arachidonic Acid Metabolism on Mucosal Integrity

2.2.1. Cyclo-oxygenase Inhibitors

Aspirin and a variety of other NSAID reduce PG synthesis by inhibiting the action of the cyclo-oxygenase enzyme. The deleterious effects of NSAID on the gastroduodenal mucosa have been well documented in animals and in human subjects. In humans, the major gastric eicosanoids are PGI_2 (prostacyclin), PGE_2, and $PGF_{2\alpha}$. While each of these PG has cytoprotective properties, PGI_2 and PGE_2 are probably the most important. It has been assumed that these compounds exert their noxious effects relative to their ability to inhibit mucosal synthesis of PG. In fact, there are experimental data both in support of and against directly relating changes in PG levels to gastric mucosal integrity. For example, significant changes in the gastric mucosal/serosal electrical potential difference (a measure of mucosal integrity) can occur without significant reduction in mucosal PG levels. Whittle (1981) showed that while a good relationship exists between PG levels and gastric damage in the rat, no such relationship was observed in the intestine following NSAID administration. His studies indicate that NSAID that are potent inhibitors of gastric mucosal PG synthesis, such as aspirin, indomethacin, flurbiprofen, and naproxen, are more damaging to the mucosa than is sodium salicylate, a weaker mucosal PG inhibitor. However, aspirin caused much more damage than did the other NSAID with comparable degrees of PG inhibition, suggesting that inhibition of PG synthesis is but one of the characteristics determining the irritant effect of certain drugs.

2.2.2. Lipoxygenase Metabolites

There is much less information available concerning the effects of the lipoxygenase (LIPO) metabolites of arachidonic acid (AA) on mucosal integrity. Theoretically, the inhibition of cyclo-oxygenase could lead to increased synthesis of LIPO metabolites as a result of less conversion of AA to PG. Maintenance of appropriate mucosal blood flow is important in preventing mucosal damage (see Chapter 8, *this volume*). Leukotriene (LT) C_4 has been reported to decrease gastric mucosal blood flow, increase pepsin secretion, and decrease gastric mucosal/serosal electrical potential difference in animals. Studies from our laboratory indicated that a LIPO inhibitor reduced ethanol-induced gastric damage in the rat. It is also possible that the LIPO hydroperoxy (hydroperoxy-eicosatetraenoic acid) metabolites of AA may interfere with the synthesis of PGI_2, an important protective eicosanoid. The administration of an NSAID could therefore set up a damaging cycle, reducing PG synthesis, increasing potentially damaging LIPO metabolites, and further reducing PGI_2 synthesis secondary to the actions of LIPO metabolities on the PGI_2 synthetic enzyme.

The potentially beneficial effects of endogenous increases in PG precursor substrates are discussed in detail in Chapter 10 (*this volume*). There are substantial data to indicate that effects on AA transformation have significant actions on the gastric mucosa and further support a regulatory role for PG in gastroduodenal mucosal integrity.

2.2.3. Cigarette Smoking

It is well known that cigarette smoking adversely affects acute ulcer healing and increases the incidence of ulcer relapses. In two differently designed clinical studies, the effect of cigarette smoking on gastric PG was assessed. In one study performed on smokers, three cigarettes smoked over a 45-min period, significantly reduced PGE_2 output in collected gastric juice. In the other study, endoscopic biopsies of gastric mucosa (fundus and antrum) and duodenum were obtained and analyzed for PGE_2 and 6-keto-$PGF_{1\alpha}$ (the stable metabolite of PGI_2) output. In this study, there were no baseline differences in PG output in nonsmokers, as compared with inactive smokers. However, smoking four cigarettes 1 hr before biopsy reduced prostanoid output in the stomach and duodenum, with a statistically significant reduction observed in the fundic biopsies where PG output was greatest.

These clinical studies in human subjects are supported by more basic research in rats in which cigarette smoke was found to decrease arachidonic acid conversion to PGI_2 in strips of aorta and increase AA conversion to thromboxane A_2 (TXA_2) in platelets. There are data to indicate that TXA_2, a potent vasoconstrictor, increases gastric mucosal damage caused by acid-dependent noxious agents. It is also interesting to note that, in these studies, the activity was limited to the particulate fraction of cigarette smoke.

It is therefore interesting to speculate that the deleterious effect of cigarette smoking on peptic ulcer disease is related to an effect on AA metabolism, further adding support for an integral role for PG in maintaining the normal mucosa.

2.3. Effects of Exogenous Prostaglandins on Mucosal Defense Mechanisms

Our current understanding of mucosal defense mechanisms is covered in detail in Chapter 4 (*this volume*). The exogenous administration of PG affects in a positive manner most of the mechanisms discussed (Table II). General nonspecific studies such as those on the gastric mucosal barrier indicate that in both animals and humans, PG administration either prevents or reduces the deleterious effects of barrier breakers, such as aspirin, ethanol, and bile acids, on the gastric mucosal barrier, as measured by changes in the negative electrical potential difference.

Prostaglandins have a number of effects on gastric mucus. Studies in animals and/or humans indicate that PG and PG analogues increase the thickness of the mucus gel layer, stimulate mucus secretion and synthesis, and change the characteristics of mucus toward a glycoprotein structure that is more resistant to acid and pepsin degradation. Recent work in our laboratories also provides

Table II. Effects of Exogenous Prostaglandin Administration

Prevent/reduce damage by barrier breakers
Increase thickness of mucus layer
Increase mucus secretion
Increase bicarbonate secretion
Maintain/increase mucosal blood flow
Stabilize tissue lysozymes/vascular endothelium
Improve mucosal regenerative capacity

evidence that PG may have a physiologic role in regulating mucosal mucus. Using cultures of gastric mucosa, we found that the inhibition of PG synthesis by indomethacin is accompanied by a fall in mucus synthesis, while stimulation of PG synthesis by exogenous AA resulted in a related increase in mucus synthesis.

Prostaglandins also increase gastric nonparietal cell secretion and duodenal bicarbonate secretion. The effect on bicarbonate secretion, observed in animals and humans, appears to be dose related and possibly to have physiologic significance. Lysosomal and vascular integrity are also improved by exogenous PG. The stabilizing effects of PG on the microvasculature may be particularly important, since it appears that one of the first abnormalities in the pathogenesis of mucosal injury is an increase in microvasculature leakiness. Finally, it has been shown in histological studies that PG limit the depth of mucosal destruction in ethanol-induced injury, permitting more rapid restitution of the damaged superficial epithelium. Indeed, a major effect of PG may be to limit rather than totally prevent mucosal damage.

2.4. Postulated Prostaglandin-Related Defects in Duodenal Ulcer Disease

2.4.1. Defects in Mucosal Defense in Duodenal Ulcer Disease

Several PG-influenced factors are believed to be important in maintaining an intact mucosa and appear to be defective in patients with duodenal ulcers, as compared with nonulcer patients.

Mucus consisting of higher-molecular-weight glycoprotein (more dense) is more resistant to acid and pepsin degradation than mucus consisting of greater concentrations of lower-molecular-weight glycoprotein (less dense). When compared with normals, patients with gastric and duodenal ulcers have been reported to have less dense mucus. Animal studies have shown that a PGE_2 analogue significantly increases the viscosity of mucus and decreases mucus degradation by pepsin. The stimulatory effects of PG on mucus synthesis, release, and resistance to degradation have recently also been described in isolated cells. Since our preliminary data indicate a relationship between mucus synthesis and PG synthesis, there is increasing evidence of a major role for PG in mucosal integrity.

It has been suggested in the past that patients with duodenal ulcers have decreased secretion of intraluminal bicarbonate, but the data are conflicting. Most of the past studies have focused on the pancreas and stomach. Studies administering indomethacin to human subjects provide conflicting data on the role of endogenous PG in regulating gastric acid and bicarbonate secretion. Some studies have reported that indomethacin increases acid secretion and decreases bicarbonate secretion, while others have failed to find such effects. Recently, a group of investigators showed in the rat that duodenal bicarbonate secretion occurs physiologically in response to acid passing through the proximal and distal duodenum and that this response appears to be under the control of endogenous PG. In these studies, inhibition of endogenous PG synthesis by pretreatment with indomethacin blocked the bicarbonate secretory response to acid—a response that was restored by the exogenous administration of PG. In a recent publication, this group has reported that the duodenal bicarbonate response to acid that they observed in rats also exists in humans. These investigators also observed that duodenal ulcer patients secreted less bicarbonate in response to duodenal acid perfusion than did nonulcer controls. Recently, it was shown that the administration of a PG analogue orally to human subjects significantly stimulates proximal and distal duodenal bicarbonate secretion.

While other postulated abnormalities in ulcer patients such as gastric emptying and duodenal–gastric reflux may be influenced by PG, very few reproducible data are available, and it will not be further pursued here. However, the data linking PG to gastroduodenal mucus secretion and structure and duodenal bicarbonate secretion are compelling.

2.4.2. Endogenous Prostaglandin Defects in Duodenal Ulcer Disease

In 1974, we postulated that a defect in gastric PG may exist in patients with duodenal ulcer disease. We observed that duodenal ulcer patients in the basal state secreted significantly less PGE into their gastric juice than did nonulcer controls and that relative to the amount of acid secreted, duodenal ulcer patients produced less PGE in both the basal and stimulated states. In 1983, other laboratories published reports indicating that the gastric and/or duodenal mucosal concentrations of several PG, primarily PGE_2 and PGI_2, were significantly less in patients with duodenal and/or gastric ulcers as compared with nonulcer controls. In one study measuring duodenal PG, no differences were found in total PG synthesized by ulcer and nonulcer subjects; however, it was observed that relative to the amount of acid perfusing the duodenum, duodenal ulcer patients produced significantly less PG than did the nonulcer controls.

While it is both difficult and risky to attempt to quantify specific factors important in the pathogenesis of an obviously multifactorial disorder such as peptic ulcer disease, at least six different laboratories have described defects in

PG synthesis and/or secretion in ulcer patients. It appears quite likely that PG act in concert with other factors in maintaining mucosal integrity and that in ulcer patients a disharmony occurs.

Recent experimental studies in rabbits immunized against prostaglandins indicated that such immunization resulted in the formation of gastric ulcers in most animals and intestinal ulcers in some of the animals. When the animals were immunized against 6-keto-$PGF_{1\alpha}$ (i.e., PGI_2) in addition to PGE_2, the number of animals that died from ulcer perforations doubled. It is hypothesized that immunization causes the production of PG antibodies, resulting in the binding of endogenous PG, thereby decreasing endogenous mucosal PG concentrations. These studies further support a role for PG in maintaining mucosal integrity.

3. THERAPEUTIC EFFECTS OF PROSTAGLANDINS ON ACUTE AND CHRONIC MUCOSAL INJURY IN HUMANS

3.1. Aspirin and NSAID-Related Injury

The clinical and experimental administration of aspirin (ASA) and other NSAID to humans results in an increased incidence of acute gastroduodenal damage (gastritis and erosions), ulcers, and bleeding. However, despite an unquestioned increase in GI symptoms, the literature does not provide clear evidence of the GI clinical risks associated with NSAID ingestion. Obviously, the patient risk of significant GI damage is extremely small. However, considering the millions of NSAID prescriptions written yearly and the vast over-the-counter (OTC) use of these drugs, the cumulative risk may indeed be great. In a recent review from the United Kingdom, 60% of patients developing a complication of ulcer disease (perforation, bleeding) were consuming NSAID, and nearly 80% of ulcer-related deaths occurred in patients taking NSAID. Moreover, the first sign of ulcer disease was a complication in nearly 60% of those taking NSAID. While much more data are needed, consensus is emerging that (1) there is probably an increased clinical incidence of gastroduodenal damage in patients taking NSAID, (2) there are reasonable data indicating that NSAID users have more ulcer complications when ulcers occur, and (3) the elderly appear to be more at risk than younger people.

In considering the effects of NSAID on the gastroduodenal mucosa, it is important to separate acute from chronic effects. A number of clinical studies have been performed looking at the gastroduodenal damaging effects of NSAID such as ASA (single dose, 1300 mg), ASA 975 mg four times daily for four days, tolmetin 400 or 500 mg four times daily for 6 days, and naproxen 500 mg twice daily for 7 days. In these studies, subjects invariably develop statistically significant increased GI bleeding (as measured by ^{51}Cr blood loss or endoscopic evidence of bleeding, gastritis or erosions. Orally administered PGE_2 or PG analogues significantly reduce this damage. In most studies, PG were effective only at dosages that also reduced acid secretion and even in studies showing efficacy at nonantisecretory dosages, increasing the dose increased the efficacy. Thus, the clear separation of a cytoprotective action from an effect on acid secretion as observed in experimental animals is not readily transposed to humans. One study compared the efficacy of cimetidine and a PGE_1 analogue on tolmetin-induced gastric damage. While both were effective in reducing damage, the PG was significantly superior to the H_2-receptor antagonist.

A recent trial investigated the efficacy of misoprostol (a PGE_1 analogue) on aspirin-induced GI damage in rheumatoid arthritis patients over a 2-month period. After 4 weeks of ASA therapy, and before patients were randomized to receive either PG or placebo, of 270 patients endoscoped 22% had ulcers, an additional 50% had discrete erosions, and only 7% were totally normal, indicating that a significant amount of gastroduodenal damage occurs during continuous ASA treatment in rheumatoid arthritis patients. Of those patients randomized, patients receiving PG showed significantly increased healing of their gastric and duodenal ulcers (75% versus 32% for the placebo group) and greater healing of all lesions (78% versus 29%) following 2 months of therapy. In addition, those patients receiving PG, in whom the mucosal damage did not totally heal showed a significant lessening of the severity of lesions present at the end of 8 weeks as compared with those receiving placebo. This study strongly suggests that the continued use of aspirin causes significant damage to the gastroduodenal mucosa and that this damage can be alleviated by the concomitant administration of a PG analogue. It was also noted that the PG-treated group of patients had no worsening of their arthritis as compared with the placebo group.

A recently completed study in osteoarthritis patients receiving Ibuprofen, Naproxen, or Piroxicam looked at the efficacy of misoprostol in preventing gastric ulceration. In the group of patients receiving placebo, the incidence of gastric ulcer was 22%, while patients receiving misoprostol 100 or 200 mg four times daily, developed a gastric ulcer 6 and 1% of the time, respectively ($p < 0.001$).

While there are several mechanisms involved in NSAID-induced mucosal damage, the preponderance of data indicates that such damage can frequently be related to the inhibitory effect of the drug on mucosal PG synthesis. Acute and chronic studies in humans show that the exogenous administration of PG can prevent or significantly reduced the damaging effects of NSAID. While PG are most effective when given at antisecretory rather than cytoprotective dosages, their superiority to H_2-receptor antagonists suggests than that PG play a unique role in maintaining the gastroduodenal mucosa.

Based upon its ability to virtually abolish NSAID-related gastric ulceration, misoprosol (Cytotec[R]) was recently approved by the U.S. Food and Drug Administration for the prevention of such damage.

3.2. Ethanol-Related Injury

Ethanol has a direct toxic effect on the gastric mucosa that does not require the presence of acid. In addition to animal work, several studies have been performed in humans to determine the protective effect of PG on ethanol-induced injury. In an endoscopically controlled study in human subjects, the efficacy of antisecretory doses of a PGE_1 analogue and cimetidine were compared with placebo with respect to preventing damage caused by spraying 40 ml 80% ethanol directly on the gastric mucosa. Significant mucosal damage occurred in those subjects receiving placebo. Both PG and cimetidine pretreatment significantly reduced the damage observed 15 and 30 min after the ethanol insult. However, PG pretreatment resulted in an almost normal mucosa and was significantly superior to cimetidine in preventing damage. Another study using normal volunteers, indicated that a PGE_2 analogue also reduced gastric and duodenal damage caused by drinking alcohol.

These studies are particularly important, considering the fact that the experimental model used is not acid dependent. They indicate that over and above their antisecretory actions, prostaglandins have an additional protective effect on the gastroduodenal mucosa.

3.3. Peptic Ulcer Disease

Over the past 10 years, a number of PGE_1 and PGE_2 analogues have been studied in controlled clinical trials, assessing their efficacy in improving acute ulcer healing. Three PGE_2 analogues (arbaprostil, enprostil, trimoprostil) and two PGE_1 analogues (misoprostol, rioprostil) have been the most extensively studied. No PG has received United States Food and Drug Administration (FDA) approval for antiulcer therapy; only misoprostol and enprostil are currently undergoing continued clinical study in the United States. Misoprostol (MISO) and enprostil (EN) have been approved for clinical use in numerous foreign countries. As has been observed with currently available standard antiulcer therapy,

PG are more effective in enhancing the healing of duodenal ulcers than gastric ulcers.

3.3.1. Gastric Ulcer—Acute Healing

There have been relatively few controlled gastric ulcer studies. A single placebo-controlled enprostil study showed EN 35 μg b.i.d. to be superior to placebo at 6 weeks (82% healing versus 52% healing), while EN 70 μg b.i.d. was not statistically superior to placebo. When enprostil was compared with ranitidine, no differences in healing efficacy were observed between the two drugs. Several placebo-controlled studies have been reported using MISO. Misoprostol 100 μg q.i.d. was found to be more effective than placebo, while MISO 25 μg b.i.d. (a nonantisecretory dose) was ineffective. When compared with cimetidine 300 mg q.i.d., MISO 50 μg q.i.d. was found to be less effective in two studies, while MISO 100 or 200 μg q.i.d. was as effective as cimetidine. In general, PG at appropriately selected dosages, are equivalent to H_2-receptor antagonists with respect to healing gastric ulcers, although the PG experience is much less than that with H_2-receptor antagonists.

3.3.2. Duodenal Ulcer—Acute Healing

A much larger number of duodenal ulcer trials have been completed. Enprostil was reported to be significantly better than placebo in healing duodenal ulcers at 4 weeks, with rates of 39%, 65%, and 78% for placebo, EN 35 μg b.i.d., and EN 70 μg b.i.d., respectively. In one study, EN 35 μg b.i.d. was comparable to cimetidine 400 mg b.i.d., while in others EN was significantly less effective than ranitidine 150 mg b.i.d. Enprostil 75 μg at night was significantly less effective than ranitidine 300 mg at night.

Misoprostol 100 and 200 μg q.i.d., as well as MISO 400 μg b.i.d., are more effective than placebo in healing duodenal ulcer at 4 weeks. In comparative trials with cimetidine, MISO 200 μg q.i.d. was as effective as cimetidine 300 mg q.i.d., while MISO 50 μg q.i.d. was less effective. In a single study, trimoprostil 750 μg q.i.d. was significantly less effective than cimetidine.

In general, average duodenal ulcer healing rates with PG are comparable to those observed with available standard ulcer therapy—40–50% at 2 weeks, and 65–85% at 4 weeks. Two important side effects are observed with PG therapy. Diarrhea has been observed in 2–25% of subjects taking PG in clinical trials. In general, the diarrhea is mild (frequently just a softening of the stool), and very few patients found it severe enough to withdraw from the studies. Preliminary data indicate that taking the PG with meals reduces the incidence and severity of diarrhea. PG analogues, at dosages as low as twice the daily therapeutic dose, may be capable of stimulating uterine contraction in pregnant women and may cause uterine emptying during the first trimester. Therefore, PG cannot be used by pregnant women or women who may become pregnant during therapy without the risk of miscarriage. There has been some concern that PG analogues would be abused by some as abortifacients. It should be pointed out that much more effective abortifacients are already available for clinical use.

3.3.3. Duodenal Ulcer Relapse

A significant problem with the long-term treatment of duodenal ulcer is the high incidence of ulcer relapse. Relapses can run in excess of 75% at 1 year in smokers, and even smokers who continue on prophylactic treatment can have 12-month relapse incidences of more than 30%. One recent study indicates that MISO therapy may overcome the deleterious effect of cigarette smoking in acute duodenal ulcer healing. A preliminary retrospective analysis of duodenal ulcer trials suggests that treatment with several nonantisecretory ulcer drugs such as bismuth subcitrate, sucralfate, and PG may be associated with fewer ulcer recurrences than that observed following treatment with H_2-receptor antagonists. Specifically, in a comparison between cimetidine and misoprostol, MISO was found to have a significantly increased time to expected ulcer recurrence (365 days) compared with that observed with cimetidine (169 days). Prospective studies are needed to confirm these retrospective observations.

4. SUMMARY

In addition to their antisecretory effects, PG have a unique ability to prevent or reduce experimental gastroduodenal mucosal damage caused by both acid-dependent and acid-independent noxious stimuli. Moreover, there are significant data to indicate that PG play a physiological role in regulating some of the endogenous mucosal defense mechanisms and that exogenous and endogenous increases in PG enhance mucosal defense. PG may also have a pathophysiological role in peptic ulcer disease, with deficiencies of PG gastroduodenal mucosal content or secretion having been described in ulcer patients. The development of stable PG analogues has made available therapy that may prove superior to conventional therapy in treating certain patients with ulcer disease, in reducing ulcer relapse, and in preventing NSAID-associated GI damage.

5. FUTURE DIRECTIONS

The evidence is overwhelming that PG play an important role in maintaining normal gastroduodenal mucosal integrity and in ameliorating mucosal damage. Future studies at the cellular level should help further define the specifics of mucosal damage as well as the PG role. While PG do not appear to offer any advantages over current therapy in the acute treatment of gastric and duodenal ulcers, several unique therapeutic possibilities require further delineation. First, it is possible that the nonhealing populations for conventional and PG-treated groups are different and that H_2-receptor nonhealers may respond better by changing to PG. Second, it is important to determine whether high-risk patients, e.g., cigarette smokers, enjoy superior healing with PG drugs. One of the most serious problems with antiulcer therapy is the high incidence of relapse; careful prospective evaluations are required to determine whether the use of certain drugs such as PG can cause a reduction in the ulcer relapse rate.

Finally, peptic ulcer complications are increased in NSAID users, particularly those over the age of 60 years. While each individual practitioner may see such complications rarely, the cumulative overall cost in terms of morbidity and mortality is significant. There are exciting new data, much as yet unpublished, suggesting that PG possess a superior ability to prevent and treat NSAID-associated gastroduodenal disease without affecting the anti-inflammatory effects of the NSAID. Additional trials are needed to corroborate the initial observations. The determination of which NSAID users should be treated with PG and what the cost–benefit characteristics of such treatment may be are additional questions that need to be answered in a complex medical/social/economic arena.

ANNOTATED BIBLIOGRAPHY

Agrawal NM, Godiwala T, Arimura A, et al: Comparative cytoprotective effects against alcohol: Misoprostol versus cimetidine. *Dig Dis Sci* **31**(suppl):142S, 1986 (abst).

The importance of this contribution is that it provides evidence for the superior effect of a prostaglandin in preventing mucosal damage when a non-acid-dependent experimental model is used.

Agrawal NM, Roth S, Mahowald M, et al: Misoprostol coadministration heals aspirin-induced gastric lesions in rheumatoid arthritis patients. *Gastroenterology* **92**:1290, 1987 (abst).

This abstract provides important data on the healing effect of a prostaglandin on gastric lesions, during continued chronic administration of aspirin. Not included in this abstract, but presented at a symposium held during Digestive Disease Week in 1987, are data showing similar (but less effective) efficacy in duodenal ulcers in this group of patients.

Ahlquist DA, Dozois RR, Zinmeister, AR, et al: Duodenal prostaglandin synthesis and acid load in health and in duodenal ulcer disease. *Gastroenterology* **85**:522–528, 1983.

In this study, the investigators did not find a significant difference between PG in the ulcer and nonulcer groups with respect to total measurements. However, they did find that ulcer patients synthesized less PG relative to the amount of acid perfusing the duodenum, thereby confirming the original work of Wilson's group.

Armstrong CP, Blower AL: Non-steroidal anti-inflammatory drugs and life threatening complication of peptic ulceration. *Gut* **28**:527–532, 1987.

This is a fairly extensive overview of NSAID-related ulcer problems in the United Kingdom. Their epidemiological data are more complete than in the United States, making this an excellent article to read.

Chaudhury TK, Robert A: Prevention by mild irritants of gastric necrosis produced in rats by sodium taurocholate. *Dig Dis Sci* **25**:830–836, 1980.

This very important article reports and details the concept of direct and adaptive cytoprotection.

Cohen, MM, Clark L, Armstrong L, et al: Reduction of aspirin-induced fecal blood loss with low-dose misoprostol tablets in man. *Dig Dis Sci* **30**:605–611, 1985.

This is one of two studies in man showing statistically significant protection against acute NSAID damage with a non-antisecretory (cytoprotective) dosage of a PG analogue.

Dickson B: Comparative incidence of ulcer relapse following treatment by misoprostol, H$_2$-antagonists and placebo. *Ital J Gastroenterol* **19**(suppl 3):21s, 1987.

This preliminary report that suggests that different antiulcer drugs may be associated with different incidences of ulcer relapse. In general, the nonantisecretory drugs had a lower relapse rate.

Graham, Dy, Agkrawal, NM, Roth, SH: Prevention of NSAID-induced gastric ulcer with misoprostol: multicenter, double-blind, placebo-controlled trial. *Lancet* **2**:1277–1280, 1988.

This is an extremely important study, providing for the first time convincing evidence that concomitant therapy can prevent NSAID-related gastric ulcer disease.

Hinsdale JG, Engel JJ, Wilson DE: Prostaglandin E in peptic ulcer disease. *Prostaglandins* **6**:495–500, 1974.

This manuscript is of historical importance, since it was the first to show a prostaglandin deficiency in ulcer disease, nearly a decade in advance of subsequent confirmation. Methodology for PG measurements was not far advanced at that time.

Isenberg JI, Smedford B, Johansson C: Effect of graded doses of intraluminal H$^+$, prostaglandin E$_2$, and inhibition of endogenous prostaglandin synthesis on proximal duodenal bicarbonate secretion in unanesthetized rat. *Gastroenterology* **88**:303–307, 1985.

This paper represents the first description of the bicarbonate physiological response to acid perfusing the duodenum and the role that endogenous and exogenous prostaglandins play in this response. It is a must.

Konturek SJ, Kwiecien N, Obtulowicz W, et al: Prostaglandins in peptic ulcer disease: Effect of nonsteroidal antiinflammatory compounds (NOSAC). *Scand J Gastroenterol* **19**(suppl 92):250–254, 1984.

This group of investigators present evidence that the degree of gastric mucosal NSAID-related damage can be readily related to the effect of the drug on prostaglandin synthesis.

Lanza FL: A double-blind study of prophylactic effect of misoprostol on lesions of gastric and duodenal mucosa induced by oral administration of tolmetin in healthy subjects. *Dig Dis Sci* **31** (suppl):131S–136S, 1986.

This representative study details the protective effect of PG analogues against NSAID-induced damage in humans. This study highlights the general observation that both damage and protection against damage are greater in the stomach than in the duodenum.

Lanza FL, Aspinall RL, Swabb EA, et al: A double-blind placebo-controlled endoscopic comparison of the cytoprotective effects of misoprostol and cimetidine on tolmetin-induced gastric mucosal injury. *Gastroenterology* **92:**1491, 1987 (abst).

This study, in abstract form, indicates that a PG analogue is superior to cimetidine in reducing or preventing tolmetin-induced gastric damage over a 7-day period. Both the PG and H_2-receptor antagonist were administered at antisecretory dosages.

Lauritsen K, Rask-Madsen J: Prostaglandins and clinical experience in peptic ulcer disease. *Scand J Gastroenterol* **21**(suppl 125):174–180, 1986.

This paper lists many of the clinical trials published by early 1986 and provides a brief overview of prostaglandin antiulcer therapy.

McQueen S, Allen A, Garner A: Measurement of gastric and duodenal mucus gel thickness, in Allen A, Flemstrom G, Garner A, Silen W, Turnberg LA (eds): *Mechanisms of Mucosal Protection in the Upper Gastrointestinal Tract.* New York, Raven, 1984, pp. 215–221.

This manuscript provides some of the initial information describing the extent of the mucus gel layer in the stomach and duodenum and details the stimulatory effects of prostaglandins and carbachol.

Quimby GF, Bonnice CA, Burstein SH: Active smoking depresses prostaglandin synthesis in human gastric mucosa. *Ann Intern Med* **104:**616–619, 1986.

Although there are some methodological problems, this brief report is the most complete study of this type done and is important to review. These investigators were the first to report this association.

Redfern JS, Blair AJ, Lee E, et al: Gastrointestinal ulcer formation in rabbits immunized with prostaglandin E_2. *Gastroenterology* **93:**744–752, 1987.

This extremely important paper shows that the theoretical reduction of endogenous PG following the induction of PG antibodies results in gastrointestinal ulceration. This is first-rate experimental evidence supporting an endogenous role for PG in ulcer pathogenesis.

Robert A: Antisecretory, anti-ulcer, cytoprotective and diarrheogenic properties of prostaglandins. *Adv Prostaglandin Thromboxane Res* **2:**507–520, 1976.

The ''real'' concept of cytoprotection is described. Robert shows that both anitsecretory and nonantisecretory PG can protect.

Robert A, Nezamis JE, Phillips JP: Effect of prostaglandin E1 on gastric secretion and ulcer formation in the rat. *Gastroenterology* **55:**481–487, 1968.

This is the first publication showing that prostaglandins can prevent experimental ulceration.

Robert A, Stowe DF, Nezamis JE: Prevention of duodenal ulcers by administration of prostaglandin E_2 (PGE$_2$). *Scand J Gastroenterol* **6:**303–305, 1971.

This article reports PG prevention of duodenal ulcers in the rat.

Robert A, Nezamis JE, Lancaster C, et al: Cytoprotection by prostaglandins in rats. Prevention of gastric necrosis produced by alcohol, HCl, NaOH, hypertonic NaCl and thermal injury. *Gastroenterology* **77**:433–443, 1979.

This manuscript details the broad effects of PG on both acid and non-acid-dependent experimental ulceration.

Selling JA, Hogan DL, Aly A, et al: Indomethacin inhibits duodenal mucosal bicarbonate secretion and endogenous prostaglandin E_2 output in human subjects. *Ann Intern Med* **106**:368–371, 1987.

In this study, the investigators extend their animal work to human studies, confirming a bicarbonate secretory response to acid in the duodenum and relating that response to endogenous prostaglandin levels.

Sharon P, Cohen F, Zifroni A, et al: Prostanoid synthesis by cultured gastric and duodenal mucosa: Possible role in the pathogenesis of duodenal ulcer. *Scand J Gastroenterol* **18**:1045–1049, 1983.

This study, using more precise techniques, reports the decreased gastric synthesis of several PG in duodenal ulcer patients. There was no difference in duodenal PG between the ulcer and nonulcer group.

Silverstein FE, Kimmey MB, Saunders DR, et al: Gastric protection by misoprostol against 1300 mg of aspirin: An endoscopic study. *Dig Dis Sci* **31**(suppl):137s–141S, 1986.

This represents one of several studies by this group showing PG protection against aspirin-induced acute damage. In later studies, these workers were able to show increasing protective efficacy with increasing dosage, followed by a plateau effect.

Szabo S, Trier JS, Brown A, et al: Early vascular injury and increased vascular permeability in gastric mucosal injury caused by ethanol in the rat. *Gastroenterology* **88**:228–236, 1985.

This important article provides a great deal of information about vascular changes in mucosal injury as well as detailing the effects of prostaglandins and sulfhydryl-containing compounds and vascular fragility and mucosal damage.

Tarnawski A, Hollander D, Stachura J, et al: Prostaglandin protection of the gastric mucosa against alcohol injury—A dynamic time-related process. *Gastroenterology* **88**:334–352, 1985.

This article is the best description of the area-specific histological effects of prostaglandins on ethanol-induced gastric necrosis. It provides specific time-related data on mucosal regeneration.

Whittle BJR: Prostaglandin–cyclo-oxygenase inhibition and its relationship to gastric damage, in Harmon JW (ed): *Basic Mechanisms of Gastrointestinal Mucosal Cell Injury and Protection.* Baltimore, William & Wilkins, 1981, pp. 197–210.

This is a brief but still relevant review of one point of view with respect to the relationship of mucosal prostaglandin levels and associated mucosal damage.

Wilson DE, Quadros E, Rajapaksa T, et al: Effects of misoprostol on gastric acid and mucus secretion in man. *Dig Dis Sci* **31**(suppl):126S–129S, 1986.

This representative article details the stimulatory effect of prostaglandin analogues on mucus secretion in humans.

10

The Role of Nutrient Essential Fatty Acids in Gastric Mucosal Protection

DANIEL HOLLANDER and ANDRZEJ TARNAWSKI

1. INTRODUCTION

Dietary therapy and nutritional manipulation have fallen into disfavor in the management of peptic ulcer disease. Before the advent of potent antacids and H_2-receptor antagonists, dietary therapy for patients with ulcer disease was very important. Patients were instructed to follow complicated rigid schemes designed to eliminate irritating foods, as these patients were placed on bland, healing diets. Patients became dietary and social cripples and were often sentenced to a lifelong adherence to dietary restriction. Fortunately, these days are over. Dietary therapy fell into oblivion because it did not work and because effective drugs appeared on the market. We certainly would not want to return to those "good old days," but recent studies from our laboratory have raised the possibility that specific dietary factors can be extremely effective in preventing mucosal injury by alcohol, aspirin, and perhaps other irritants. These protective dietary factors are the two essential fatty acids—arachidonic and linoleic and related fatty acids.

DANIEL HOLLANDER • Division of Gastroenterology, Department of Medicine, University of California–Irvine, Irvine, California 92717. ANDRZEJ TARNAWSKI • Veterans Administration Medical Center, Long Beach, California 90822; and Division of Gastroenterology, Department of Medicine, University of California–Irvine, Irvine, California 92717.

2. DIETARY PRECURSORS OF PROSTANOID SYNTHESIS

The gastroduodenal mucosa and most other tissues synthesize prostanoids from arachidonic or linoleic acids. Normally, arachidonic acid is stored in cell membranes as a phospholipid. Background endogenous synthesis of prostaglandins (PG) is derived from the circulating metabolic pool of essential fatty acids (EFA), while stimulated synthesis (such as in trauma or irritation) comes from the cell membrane pool. In the latter process, the enzyme phospholipase A_2 releases arachidonic acid from the cell membrane and provides the fatty acid for prostanoid synthesis through the cyclo-oxygenase or lipoxygenase pathways (for greater detail, see Chapter 9). The most common dietary EFA is linoleic acid, which is present in significant amounts in vegetable oils such as corn or safflower oil. Once ingested, linoleic acid can be used directly as a caloric source or can be metabolized into PG. If present in amounts beyond the immediate needs, linoleic acid can be converted by most tissues into arachidonic acid and stored in cell membranes as a phospholipid. This occurs in most mammals, including humans. Carnivorous animals are unable to convert linoleic acid to arachidonic acid and therefore have to eat meat or liver as arachidonic acid sources.

Prostanoids can also be synthesized from fatty acids not usually found in the Western diet. Evening primrose oil is rich in γ-linoleic acid, which can be converted to PG. Omega-3 fatty acids are fatty acids present in fish oils that can be converted predominantly into biologically inactive thromboxanes but biologically active prostaglandins (the PGI series).

3. PROTECTIVE ACTIVITY OF DIETARY ESSENTIAL FATTY ACIDS AGAINST ACUTE INJURY

The first experiments to demonstrate the efficacy of dietary EFA in protecting the gastric mucosa against alcohol injury were done in our laboratory using solubilized arachidonic acid. Normally, arachidonic acid is absorbed by the jejunum by a process that requires the presence of biological detergents such as bile acids. In order to solubilize arachidonic acid and make it available for absorption by the gastric mucosal cells, we dissolved it with a nonionic detergent—pluronic F-68. This form of arachidonic acid, when given to rats by gavage, caused a rapid synthesis of prostaglandin E_2 (PGE_2) with a several thousand-fold increase in its lumenal concentration within a short time (30 min). When we pretreated rats with solubilized arachidonic or linoleic acids, we were able to prevent (>98%) gastric mucosal damage by alcohol and aspirin (see Figs.

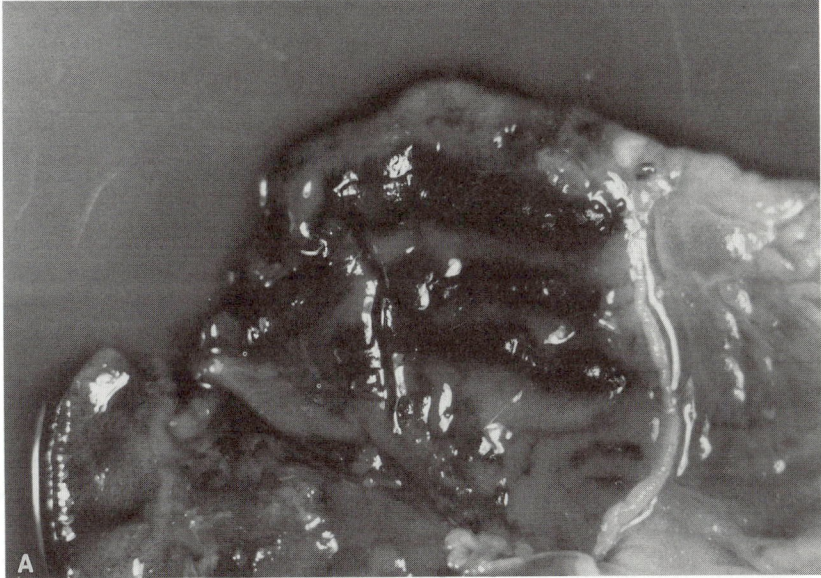

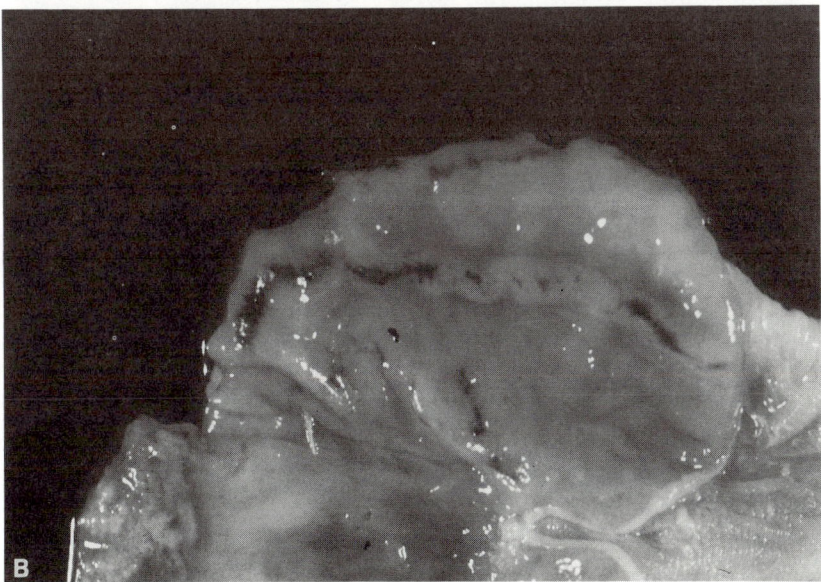

Figure 1. Gross appearance of rat gastric mucosa 3 hr after alcohol administration. (A) Saline- or solubilizer-pretreated rats. Longitudinal, necrotic, hemorrhagic lesions are present. (B) Stomach of rats pretreated with solubilized arachidonic acid. Hemorrhagic necrotic lesions are minimized by fatty acid preadministration.

1 and 2). By pretreating the rats with indomethacin in order to block the conversion of arachidonic acid to PG, we were able to abolish 60–70% of the protective activity of EFA. These experiments demonstrate that dietary EFA are extremely effective in protecting the gastric mucosa against acute injury. EFA protect the mucosa by conversion to prostanoids by mucosal enzymes. The most recent studies demonstrated that in addition to their protective action, EFA (arachidonic and linoleic), given as a treatment, exert trophic and angiogenic effects on established mucosal injury.

4. ADVANTAGES OF DIETARY ESSENTIAL FATTY ACIDS OVER SYNTHETIC PROSTAGLANDINS

The obvious question to be answered is: Why should we investigate dietary fatty acids as protective agents if synthetic prostanoids are available? Since pharmaceuticals companies have already produced potent synthetic analogues of natural PG, why should we consider using dietary fatty acids as PG precursors?

The overwhelming reason for developing therapeutic uses for dietary EFA is the rapid degradation of their natural PG products and therefore the lack of side effects from their generation compared with the side effects of the synthetic PG analogues. Natural PG have a short biological half-life. When produced by the gastric mucosa, natural PG enter the portal circulation and are removed and deactivated during their first pass through the liver and/or lungs. Thus, natural PG generated by the gastric mucosa from dietary EFA do not reach the systemic circulation and therefore are not associated with systemic side effects.

By contrast, the structure of synthetic PG analogues has been modified by methyl group additions to various portions of the molecule. These structural modifications were introduced in order to stabilize these analogues. Unfortunately, this has also resulted in the inability of the enzyme systems in liver and lung tissues to degrade and metabolize the synthetic analogues resulting in the prolonged systemic circulation of these potent compounds, causing a wide gamut of side effects, which includes diarrhea, abdominal cramps, changes in bone metabolism, uterine contractions, and even abortions.

The side effects of the PG synthetic analogues do not occur with natural PG synthesized by the gastric mucosa after the administration of dietary EFA because of the rapid degradation and removal of these prostanoids by the liver and lungs. Therefore, if dietary EFA can be administered orally with the appropriate detergent molecule, they may provide us with the ideal mucosal protective prop-

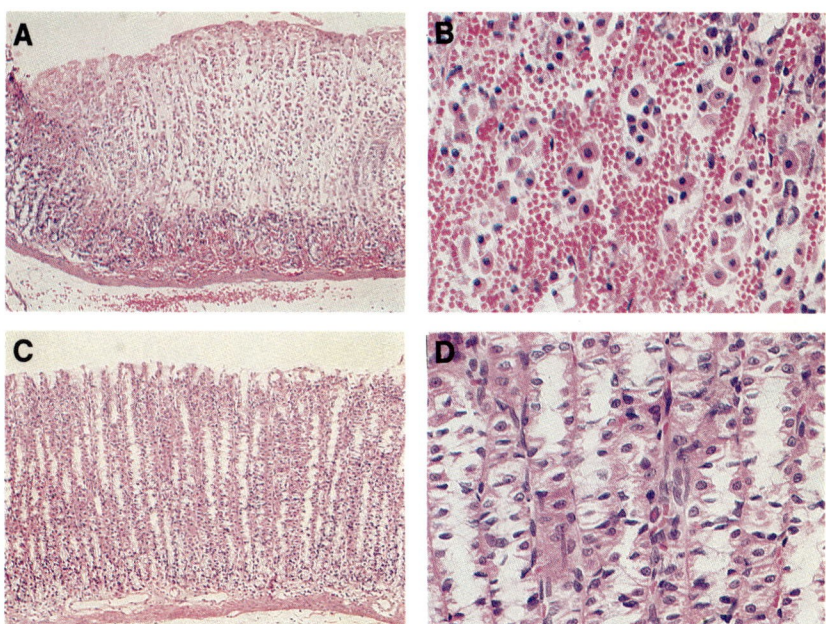

Figure 2. Histology of rat gastric mucosa. Specimens were stained with H & E. (A) Deep erosions were present 3 hr after alcohol administration in rats pretreated with solubilizer. (x100) (B) Ruptured gastric mucosal microvessels and extensive red blood cell extravasation were seen in and around the erosions. Microvascular changes precede and are the most likely cause of necrotic lesions. (x400) (C) Gastric mucosa of a rat pretreated with arachidonic acid and injured with alcohol. (x100) The mucosa is preserved without erosions or necrosis. (D) Higher-power appearance of the mucosa in rat pretreated with arachidonic acid and injured with alcohol. (x400) Fatty acid pretreatment resulted in preservation of the mucosa and mucosal microvessels.

erties and at the same time do not produce the systemic side effects of the synthetic PG analogues.

5. MUCOSAL PROTECTIVE EFFECT OF CHRONIC FEEDING OF DIETARY ESSENTIAL FATTY ACIDS

Schepp and co-workers tested the influence of dietary linoleic acid on gastric mucosal resistance to injury by 6-week feeding of groups of rats with deficient (0.3%), sufficient (3%), and supplemented (10%) diets with linoleic acid. After 6 weeks, these investigators found that the extent of gastric mucosal injury by cold restraint was inversely related to the amount of linoleic acid in the diet. The highest amount of injury was seen in rats fed a linoleic acid-deficient diet (0.3%), while injury was minimal in rats fed a 10% linoleic acid-supplemented diet. The amount of PG in the gastric lumen and in the mucosa was the highest in rats fed 10% linoleic acid. These experiments clearly demonstrate that chronic dietary deficiency of linoleic acid predisposes rats to gastric mucosal injury, while dietary supplementation with linoleic acid was effective in reducing mucosal injury. These studies are very important in demonstrating that chronic feeding of dietary EFA can greatly affect mucosal resistance to injury after 6 weeks of dietary modification. On the basis of this study, we propose that the long-term dietary supply of EFA could be an important determinant of the resistance of the gastroduodenal mucosa to injury.

6. EFFECT OF DIETARY ESSENTIAL FATTY ACIDS ON HUMAN GASTRIC MUCOSA

Thus far, experimental information about the effects of dietary EFAs on the human stomach are extremely limited. In a study by Grant and co-workers, this question was examined in normal male volunteers who took 1 g linoleic acid with Pluronic F-68 detergent twice daily for 2 weeks. At the end of the study, these volunteers were found to have a small reduction in their basal and stimulated acid output, a significant rise in serum gastrin, and a pronounced increase in their intragastric content of PG. This study demonstrates that the solubilized form of linoleic acid can induce functional changes in the human stomach compatible with the generation of endogenous PG. It remains to be seen whether the increased generation of PG will protect the human gastric mucosa against injury or promote the healing of established injury.

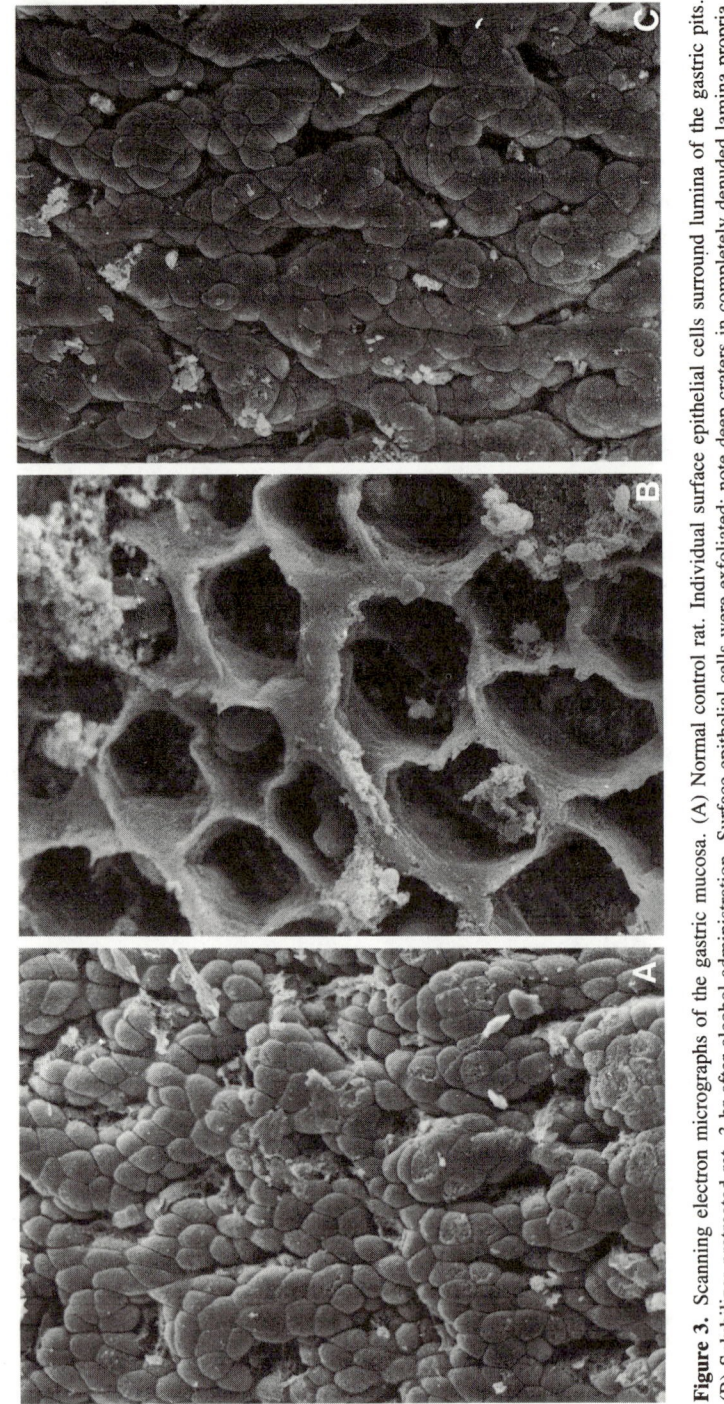

Figure 3. Scanning electron micrographs of the gastric mucosa. (A) Normal control rat. Individual surface epithelial cells surround lumina of the gastric pits. (B) Solubilizer-pretreated rat, 3 hr after alcohol administration. Surface epithelial cells were exfoliated; note deep craters in completely denuded lamina propria. (C) Rats pretreated with arachidonic or linoleic acid, at 3 hr after alcohol; restored surface epithelial cells cover the mucosal surface. (x900)

7. DIETARY ESSENTIAL FATTY ACIDS AND THE EPIDEMIOLOGY OF PEPTIC ULCER DISEASE

In order to evaluate the importance of dietary EFA in peptic ulcer disease, we collected data about dietary EFA intake in the United States and in the United Kingdom during the past 70 years. Because dietary histories or dietary recall are notoriously inaccurate, we obtained information from the U.S. Department of Agriculture about total population consumption of dietary EFA for each decade. We obtained similar data from the United Kingdom. It became apparent from the data that, during the past 70 years, there has been a slight (2–3%) decrease in the consumption of saturated EFA. Most surprisingly, however, the consumption of linoleic acid, the major dietary PG precursor, increased by approximately 200%. Since the consumption of linoleic acid by experimental animals or humans does result in higher PG synthesis, theoretically we should be finding a concomitant increase in gastric mucosal resistance. This hypothesis is amply supported by the well-documented decrease in peptic ulcer mortality, hospitalization, and operative rate that has been taking place during the past 70 years both in Europe and in the United States. This epidemiological analysis supports the hypothesis that increased dietary intake of PG precursor EFA did indeed correlate with population-wide decrease in the incidence and virulence of peptic ulcer disease in the Western world. Furthermore, this analysis suggests that the concept of cytoprotection may apply to long-term changes in gastric mucosal resistance to injury by entire populations. Thus, this concept may well apply to situations that are not limited to acute mucosal protection.

8. CONCLUSIONS AND FUTURE DIRECTIONS

We now have conclusive evidence that the two dietary EFA, arachidonic and linoleic acid, can protect the gastric mucosa of experimental animals against acute injury. We also know that these fatty acids can induce the human gastric mucosa to produce PG. Chronic feeding experiments in rats demonstrate that dietary supplementation with EFA results in increased gastric mucosal resistance to injury. Furthermore, we have epidemiological evidence that one of the causes for the decrease in ulcer incidence and virulence is the population-wide 200% increase in linoleic acid consumption over the past 50–70 years. Clearly, dietary EFA are important in promoting mucosal resistance to injury, and perhaps in decreasing the incidence and virulence of peptic ulcer disease.

What are the future implications of these new findings? The crystal ball is not entirely clear, but some distinct future developments should be mentioned. It is very possible that we may have a clear scientifically supportable reason for suggesting a dietary therapeutic program for patients with chronic peptic disease. These patients could well benefit from dietary supplementation with linoleic acid or arachidonic acid. Before we embark on such recommendations, we will need to conduct prospective trials of dietary supplementation with EFA in carefully selected patient populations.

The second major crystal ball conclusion could be the use of detergent-solubilized EFA in treating active peptic disease. The major reason for exploring this possibility is the safety of generating endogenous PG and their possible efficacy. Because of the inherent lack of systemic side effects and toxicity of endogenous PG, as compared with synthetic PG analogues, therapeutic trials of peptic ulcer patients with solubilized EFA are warranted.

ANNOTATED BIBLIOGRAPHY

Crawford MA: Background to EFA and their prostanoid derivatives. *Br Med Bull* **39**:210–213, 1983.

> This is an excellent review of biological role of essential fatty acids with a special focus on their role as prostaglandin precursors.

Grant HW, Palmer KR, Kelly RW, et al: Dietary linoleic acid, gastric acid and prostaglandin secretion. *Gastroenterology* **94**:955–959, 1988.

> This paper demonstrates that solubilized linoleic acid increases gastric luminal prostaglandins concentration and inhibits acid secretion in normal human volunteers.

Hollander D, Tarnawski A: Dietary essential fatty acids and the decline in peptic ulcer disease—A hypothesis. *Gut* **27**:239–242, 1986.

> This paper presents a hypothesis linking consumption of dietary essential fatty acids and decline in peptic ulcer disease.

Hollander D, Tarnawski A, Ivey KJ, et al: Arachidonic acid protection of rat gastric mucosa against ethanol injury. *J Lab Clin Med* **100**:286–308, 1982.

> This paper demonstrated for the first time the protective action of arachidonic acid against necrotizing agent (ethanol) injury of the gastric mucosa in an animal model.

Schepp W, Steffen B, Ruoff HJ, et al: Modulation of rat gastric mucosal prostaglandin E_2 release by dietary linoleic acid: effect on gastric acid secretion and stress-induced mucosal damage. *Gastroenterology* **95**:18–25, 1988.

> These investigators found that a long-term diet rich in linoleic acid reduced gastric acid secretion, stimulated gastric generation of prostaglandin E_2, and reduced formation of the stress ulcers in rats. A diet deficient in linoleic acid had the opposite effect.

Tarnawski A, Hollander D, Stachura J, et al: Arachidonic acid protection of gastric mucosa against alcohol injury: Sequential analysis of morphologic and functional changes. *J Lab Clin Med* **102**:34–51, 1983.

This paper explores the time sequence of morphological and functional protection of the gastric mucosa by arachidonic acid against ethanol injury in a rat model.

Tarnawski A, Hollander D, Gergely H: Protection of the gastric mucosa by linoleic acid—A nutrient essential fatty acid. *Clin Invest Med* **10:**132–136, 1987.

This paper provides experimental evidence that solubilized linoleic acid is also able to protect the gastric mucosa against ethanol injury in the rat.

11

Gastroprotection by Nonprostaglandin Substances

STANISLAW J. KONTUREK and JAN W. KONTUREK

1. INTRODUCTION

Cytoprotection is the term originally introduced into gastrointestinal (GI) pathophysiology by Robert to describe the unique feature of prostaglandins (PG) to prevent acute necrotic lesions of the GI mucosa at nonantisecretory doses. This phenomenon has been studied extensively, primarily in experimental animals, and two major categories of cytoprotection have been identified: direct cytoprotection induced by PG administered exogenously, and adaptive cytoprotection elicited by mild irritants and probably mediated by endogenous PG. Since histologic examination of the PG-protected mucosa reveals that only deep hemorrhagic necrosis is prevented—the surface epithelium becomes damaged—the term cytoprotection has been questioned. Although the surface epithelium cells are lost, the prevention by PG of deep hemorrhagic necrosis and of damage to the cells around the mucous neck allows for rapid cell migration and restitution of the integrity of surface epithelium and almost complete preservation of organ functions. The use of organoprotection (e.g., gastroprotection) is now recommended and is reviewed in this chapter.

Gastrointestinal mucosa is capable of generating not only protective PG, but also several damaging prostanoids, such as platelet-activating factor (PAF),

STANISLAW J. KONTUREK and JAN W. KONTUREK • Institute of Physiology, Academy of Medicine, 31-531 Krakow, Poland.

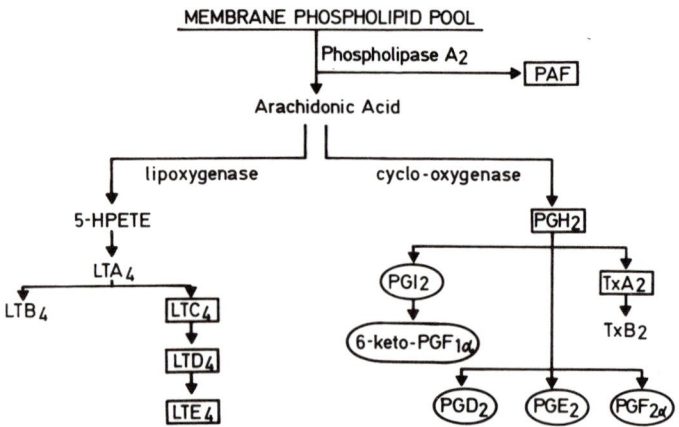

Figure 1. Biosynthetic scheme of arachidonate metabolism with products considered to be putative mediators of gastroprotection (in circles) and of ischemia and tissue damage (in boxes).

thromboxanes (Tx), and products of the lipoxygenase pathway, i.e., leukotrienes (LT). These lipid mediators derived from the arachidonate cascade have deleterious actions on gastric microcirculation and mucosal integrity. Pharmacological modulation of their release and action results in the decrease of gastric damage induced by certain ulcerogens (Fig. 1).

In addition to PG, the first endogenous compounds implicated in gastroprotection, many other endogenous substances not related to PG have been shown to prevent acute gastric mucosal injury. The list of these endogenous non-PG mucosal protectors includes endogenous sulfhydryls (SH) and certain gut hormones, e.g., epidermal growth factor (EGF), gastrin, and somatostatin.

Although chronic peptic ulcerations represent localized deep defects extending through the muscularis mucosae, obviously differing from diffuse acute mucosal damage generally used in studies on gastroprotection, major efforts have been undertaken to reinvestigate the old and new antiulcer drugs for their possible gastroprotective activity. All three classes of antiulcer drugs—the classic antisecretory drugs (anticholinergics, H_2-blockers, proton pump inhibitors), antacids, and agents that coat and protect the mucosa (carbenoxolone, Solon, colloidal bismuth subcitrate, and sucralfate)—have been reported to exhibit various degrees of gastroprotection (Guth, 1987). The last two classes were found to be the most efficacious in gastroprotection, hence are termed gastroprotective antiulcer agents. Some of these agents are believed to act, at least in part, by increasing mucosal generation of endogenous PG (Konturek, 1986).

Several other non-PG gastroprotective compounds such as sulfhydryl agents, including substances containing inorganic zinc, copper, and selenium, as well as blockers of biosynthesis of endogenous histamine, were found in certain experimental conditions to protect the gastric mucosa against noxious agents.

The concept of gastroprotection was originally developed from studies in experimental animals. Then both PG, particularly their methylated analogues, and gastroprotective drugs were successfully examined in humans for their ability to protect against certain types of mucosal damage, such as that induced by nonsteroidal anti-inflammatory drugs (NSAID) or ethanol. This chapter focuses on gastroprotection by non-PG substances and drugs and reviews their possible mechanisms of action.

2. GASTROPROTECTION BY SUPPRESSION OF RELEASE OR ACTION OF PAF, TX, OR LT IN THE GASTRIC MUCOSA

The gastric mucosa synthesizes and releases significant quantities of various vasoactive eicosanoids, which are the products of arachidonate metabolism through the cyclo-oxygenase pathway. These compounds are crucial for maintaining adequate vascular perfusion and mucosal integrity. The same enzyme, phospholipase A_2, which releases the eicosanoid precursor, arachidonic acid, is also involved in the liberation of PAF, a low-molecular-weight phospholipid that can be formed by a variety of cell types, including macrophages, neutrophils, and endothelial cells. Systemic release of PAF may contribute to the circulatory changes in endotoxic and septic shock. Wallace and Whittle (1986) showed that intravenous infusion of PAF at the dose that raised blood levels of this lipid mediator during endotoxemia induced damage of gastric mucosa in rats as a result of extensive vasocongestion, deep mucosal necrosis, and hemorrhage. This effect was not a consequence of local release of TxA_2 from the platelets, as it could not be prevented by indomethacin—a potent inhibitor of the cyclo-oxygenase pathway—or by the depletion of platelets. The most characteristic feature of PAF is pro-ulcerogenic activity and the ability to augment mucosal damage provoked by other irritants, such as ethanol, aspirin, or taurocholate. This effect appears to be specific because potent stable analogues of PGE_2, such as 16,16-dimethyl PGE_2 ($dmPGE_2$), which completely protected the mucosa against ethanol damage, failed to prevent gastric injury induced by PAF. By contrast, the specific antagonism of PAF receptors by substances (e.g., BN 52021) extracted by Braquet et al. (1988) from a crude Ginkgo biloba, almost completely prevented PAF-induced mucosal lesions or PAF-augmented gastric

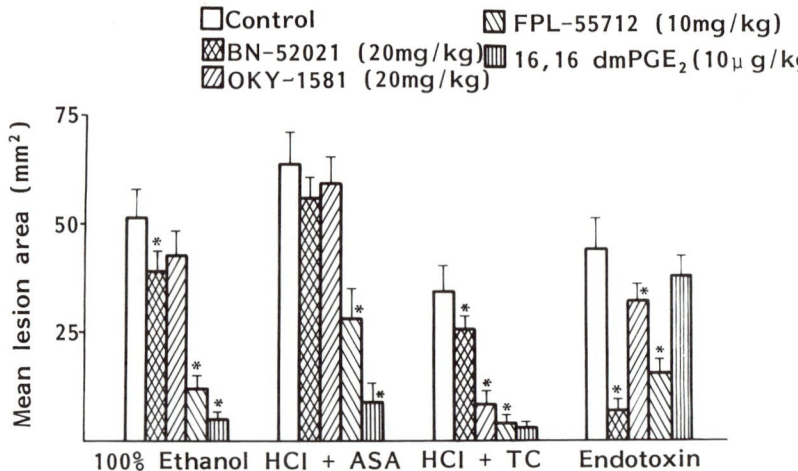

Figure 2. Gastric lesions induced in rats by intragastric administration of 100% ethanol, acidified aspirin (ASA) (200 mg/kg), acidified 100 mM taurocholate (TC), or intravenous endotoxin (10 mg/kg) alone (control), with pretreatment with PAF antagonist BN-52021 (20 mg/kg), thromboxane synthesis inhibitor OKY-1581 (20 mg/g), LTC$_4$ antagonist FPL 55712 (10 mg/kg), or 16,16-dimethyl PGE$_2$ (10 μg/kg). Means ±SEM of at least 10 rats per group. Asterisk (*) indicates significant decrease below the lesion area obtained with ulcerogen alone.

damage caused by ethanol, aspirin, or restraint stress. It is of interest that PAF may be the major mediator of GI damage induced by endotoxin because PAF antagonists afforded nearly complete protection against this damage. These studies clearly demonstrate that PAF may play a major role in the gastric mucosal damage by endotoxin and may contribute to the gastric lesions induced by ethanol, aspirin, or stress. These studies also indicate a potential therapeutic use of PAF antagonists for certain types of GI lesions, particularly those occurring in endotoxic shock and necrotizing enterocolitis, where PG are ineffective. Pretreatment with the PAF antagonist (BN-52021) had little influence on ethanol-, aspirin-, or taurocholate-induced gastric lesions but protected the mucosa against endotoxin-induced injury that was not affected by 16,16 dmPGE$_2$ (Fig. 2).

Not all eicosanoids exert a protective effect on the gastric mucosa. TxA$_2$ is a potent vasoconstrictor of blood vessels and an aggregator of platelets. Although TxA$_2$ has a very short half-life, its effect is amplified by the fact that it aggregates platelets and constricts blood vessels that trap additional platelets locally. Also, TxA$_2$ is released from aggregating platelets and in turn triggers the release of TxA_2 from other uninvolved platelets. This process may cause temporal as well as spatial augmentation of the effects of TxA_2 to be more severe than one would expect from its very short half-life.

Whittle and Vane (1987) reported that local vasoconstriction induced by Tx generated from arachidonic acid (AA) injected into the gastric artery greatly enhanced the damage induced by acidified taurocholate in the canine fundic mucosa. Mucosal damage similar to that induced by TxA_2 generated *in situ* was also obtained by its stable epoxymethanomimetic, U-46619, a potent vasoconstrictive agent. We (Konturek *et al.*, 1983) found that the rat oxyntic mucosa was capable of generating marked amounts of TxA_2. We also found that the inhibition of TxA_2 biosynthesis by the administration of specific inhibitors resulted in increase in the PGE_2 and PGI_2 formation probably because of the availability of greater amounts of substrate for PG biosynthesis. Tx inhibitors such as OKY-1581 or OKY 046 protected the gastric mucosa against the damage induced mainly by acidified taurocholate, but not by absolute ethanol, aspirin, or endotoxin (see Fig. 2). Therefore, we postulated that these beneficial effects of Tx inhibitors could be attributed to the suppression of the formation of vasoconstrictive TxA_2 and to the redirection of endoperoxide substrate to protective PGI_2 and PGE_2 in the mucosa. These studies indicate that TxA_2 may be an important mediator of mucosal ischemia, contributing significantly to the pathophysiology of acute gastric damage induced by bile salts; inhibition of TxA_2 formation by specific inhibitors may be clinically useful in the prevention of certain types of acute mucosal damage.

Another potent vasoconstrictors generated by the gastric mucosa are LT, particularly LTC_4 and LTD_4, recently identified in the gastric mucosa, particularly following exposure to ethanol or aspirin damage. LT are produced by a host of cell types, including macrophages, mast cells, leukocytes, and connective tissue cells under the influence of proinflammatory substances (e.g., PAF, stress, or ethanol). LT may also trigger the release of other mediators, such as TxA_2, which then may cause tissue damage.

Leukotrienes exert a variety of biological actions that could contribute to their role as mediators of ischemia and tissue damage (Konturek *et al.*, 1988). LTB_4 promotes the release of lysosomal hydrolases accompanied by enhancement of microvascular permeability. The peptides LTC_4 and LTD_4, are more active as stimulators of smooth muscle contraction causing marked vasoconstriction. Using *in vivo* microscopy technique to study gastric submucosal arteriolar and venular responses, Whittle and Vane (1987) observed that topical application of LTC_4 in 25–400 mM concentrations induced a marked vasoconstriction that was more extensive in venules than in arterioles, resulting in sluggish blood flow, stasis, mucosal ischemia, and tissue damage. Peskar *et al.* (1986) reported recently that gastric mucosa generates significant amounts of LTC_4, particularly when exposed to ethanol damage. It has been suggested that LTC_4 contributes to the mucosal damage by ethanol through mucosal vasocongestion and the plasma leakage from the vascular bed. Inhibition of LTC_4 formation by carbenoxolone resulted in partial reduction of gastric damage.

We found that LTC_4, when given intravenously, caused a potent vasoconstriction in the gastric mucosa and greatly enhanced the mucosal damage induced by ethanol, aspirin, taurocholate, or restraint–stress in rats. All these pro-ulcerogenic effects of exogenous LTC_4 can be suppressed by specific antagonists of LTC receptors, such as FPL 55712, which also effectively reduced the extent of acute gastric damage by various necrotizing substances (see Fig. 2). It is of interest that the lipoxygenase inhibitors such as nordihydroguaiaretic acid (NDGA) or the antiulcer drug carbenoxolone, which reduced tissue level of LTC_4, also protected the mucosa against damage induced by various irritants, particularly by ethanol, PAF, aspirin, and restraint–stress. Thus, the suppression of tissue biosynthesis or the action of endogenous LT may provide new approaches to the prevention or treatment of acute mcosal damage involving non-PG arachidonate metabolites via the lipoxygenase pathway.

3. ENDOGENOUS NONPROSTAGLANDIN GASTROPROTECTIVE SUBSTANCES: SULFHYDRYLS, EGF, GASTRIN, SOMATOSTATIN

The GI tract is the largest endocrine organ of the body, producing a great number of biologically active peptides that function either as circulating hormones (e.g., gastrin, CCK, or secretin) or as paracrine hormones that act locally in the tissue (e.g., somatostatin) or are released into the gut lumen (e.g., EGF). Some of these peptides have been shown to protect the gastric mucosa against certain types of the mucosal injury partly by affecting the balance between forces acting to destroy the lining of the GI tract and those acting to maintain it or rebuild it (Konturek *et al.*, 1982). The destructive forces, such as bile salts, stress, ethanol, or aspirin, are known to decrease the rate of mucosal cell proliferation and DNA synthesis as well as to destroy the lining by direct necrotizing actions on the mucosal cells.

Among the gut peptides, which are best known to stimulate mucosal growth and to maintain mucosal integrity, EGF and gastrin are effective in the attenuation of certain types of tissue damage, such as that induced by aspirin or restraint stress. The mechanism of this protection has not been explained, but the stimulation of polyamine synthesis by activation of ornithidine decarboxylase may play a significant role in mucosal protection from further injury, because polyamines are required for mucosal growth.

Epidermal growth factor (Gregory, 1975) is a polypeptide containing 53 amino acids. Structurally, it resembles urogastrone, another peptide that was shown several decades before to exhibit beneficial effects on healing of chronic ulcerations occurring at a dose range incapable of affecting gastric acid secretion. Both EGF and urogastrone are potent mitogens both *in vivo* and *in vitro*, their growth-promoting action being mediated by increased polyamine synthesis in gastric epithelial cells.

The major sources of EGF are salivary, pancreatic, and Brunner's glands. EGF enters the gut lumen in large amounts with salivary and duodenal secretions. Since luminal EGF is quite resistant to degradation by gastric proteases and is not absorbed by the intestine, luminal EGF may play an important physiological role in stimulating cell proliferation and in maintaining the integrity of GI mucosa.

The importance of EGF in the protective mechanism and mucosal integrity has been supported by several studies. We reported that exogenous EGF prevents aspirin-induced gastric ulcerations dose-dependently; it was at least as effective as PG but had no influence on the biosynthesis of endogenous PG (Fig. 3). Similarly, Olsen *et al.* (1984) demonstrated that saliva-containing EGF and EGF

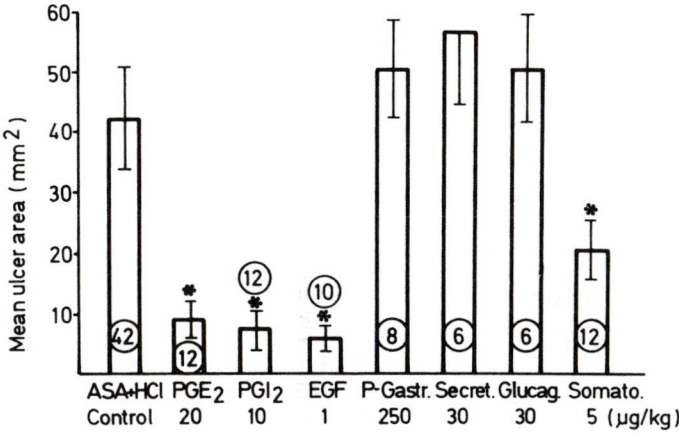

Figure 3. Effects of the pretreatment with various gut peptides on mean gastric ulcer area induced by intragastric acidified aspirin (ASA). For comparison, the effects of PGE_2 and PGI_2 are included. All tested peptides or PG were administered subcutaneously 30 min before acidified ASA. Figures in circles indicate the number of rats used in each experimental group. Asterisk (*) indicates significant ($p < 0.05$) decrease below the control value obtained with acidified ASA alone.

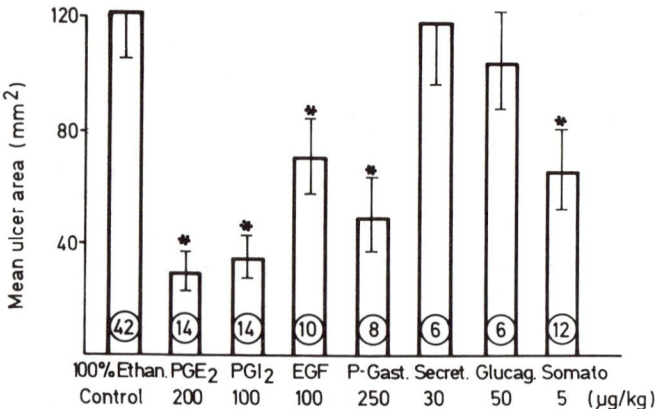

Figure 4. Effects of pretreatment with various gut peptides on acute gastric mucosal damage induced by absolute ethanol. For comparison, the effects of PGE_2 or PGI_2 are included. Figures in circles indicate the number of animals used in each experimental group. Means $\pm$SEM. Asterisk (*) indicates significant ($p < 0.05$) reduction below the value obtained with ethanol alone.

itself in nonantisecretory doses protected the mucosa against cysteamine-induced lesions and that removal of submandibular glands prompted the formation of duodenal ulcerations by cysteamine. EGF was less effective, however, in the prevention of mucosal damage caused by necrotizing agents such as absolute ethanol, which is frequently used in studies of gastric cytoprotection (Fig. 4). The inefficacy of EGF against ethanol damage may be due to the mechanisms of EGF protective activity. EGF appears to stimulate polyamine synthesis, which then results in stimulation of mucosal proliferation. Since this chain of events takes time, EGF is probably less effective against rapidly injurious agents such as ethanol. In the models of more prolonged formation of gastric lesions such as these (using acidified aspirin or cysteamine), EGF-induced protection is effective. Indeed, we observed that EGF prevented the decrease in mucosal DNA synthesis and the reduction in DNA and RNA content caused by aspirin or by restraint–stress. This protection by EGF was followed by attenuation of the gastric ulceration formation.

Similar prevention of aspirin- and stress-induced ulcerations could be achieved by the prior administration of other trophic hormones, such as gastrin and growth hormone. This prevention was closely correlated with increased DNA synthesis. As shown by Takeuchi and Johnson (1982), using rats depleted of gastrin by prolonged maintenance on a liquid diet, the reduction in DNA synthesis in the oxyntic mucosa greatly increased the ulcerogenicity of restraint–stress. Treatment with pentagastrin, which reversed the effects of liquid diet on

DNA synthesis, protected significantly against stress ulcerations, suggesting that the strengthening of regenerative forces of the gastric mucosa may be an important protective mechanism. Pentagastrin also reduced aspirin-induced gastric lesions, particularly in gastrin-depleted animals. A positive significant correlation was found between the ulcer index and the ratio of DNA loss to DNA synthesis. Again, the decreased mucosal proliferative capacity by gastrin depletion was associated with increased aspirin-induced damage; this was reversed, in part, by increased cell proliferation, using exogenous gastrin.

It is of interest that the mucosal growth-promoting effects of EGF, growth hormone, or gastrin not only may contribute to the prevention of acute gastric lesions (aspirin, restraint stress) but may also enhance healing of experimentally induced chronic gastroduodenal ulcerations (Fig. 5) (Konturek *et al.*, 1988). The removal of salivary glands (to reduced endogenous sources of EGF) or the depletion of gastrin by keeping animals on a liquid diet reduced the healing rate of chronic ulcerations remarkably; this could be reversed by administration of oral EGF or by injection of gastrin. The delay in ulcer healing in EGF- or gastrin-depleted animals was accompanied by a reduction in DNA synthesis and total DNA and RNA content in the gastric mucosa. All these biochemical indices of mucosal growth were returned to normal by pretreatment with EGF or pentagastrin. This finding reinforces the concept that mucosal cell proliferation stimulated by growth-promoting factors such as EGF or gastrin is an important factor in healing of gastroduodenal ulcerations.

Somatostatin, which is present in the endocrine–paracrine cells and in the

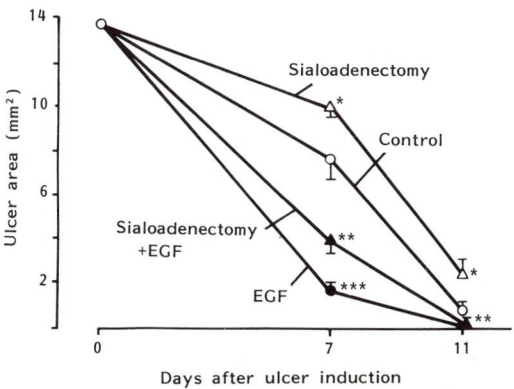

Figure 5. Chronic gastric ulcerations induced by serosal application of acetic acid on the area of 13.8 mm^2 after 7 and 11 days in rats with intact (control) and resected submandibulary glands, without and with subcutaneous treatment with EGF (30 µg/kg per day). Each point is the mean (±SEM) of at least 10 rats. Single asterisk (*) indicates significant ($p < 0.05$) increase above the control value. Double asterisk (**) indicate significant decrease below the control value obtained in rats with intact salivary glands. Triple asterisk (***) indicate significant decrease below the value obtained in rats with resected salivary glands and treated with EGF.

autonomic nerves of the gut, is known to suppress the release of other gut hormones, especially gastrin, yet it also exhibits antiulcer and gastroprotective effects. Somatostatin is highly effective in the prevention of acute gastric or duodenal lesions induced by stress, cysteamine, aspirin, and, to some extent, ethanol (see Figs. 3 and 4). Somatostatin protection against some of these lesions (stress, aspirin, cysteamine) could simply be attributed to the inhibition of gastric acid secretion, but other mechanisms, such as replacement of mucosal peptides required to reduce duodenal motility (cysteamine ulcerations) or the influence on mucosal blood flow, may also be implicated. It is of interest that the well-recognized antitrophic effects of somatostatin on the gastroduodenal mucosa do not appear to interfere with the gastroprotection by somatostatin.

Natural somatostatins with 14- or 28-amino acid residues have short-lived effects; therefore, for practical reasons, more potent cyclic analogues are now used. They have higher protective efficacy and prolonged protective action against various forms of mucosal damage such as that caused by ethanol or aspirin in experimental animals. Long-acting somatostatin analogues have been successfully used in therapy of patients with acute gastric bleeding, probably due to suppression of gastric secretion and decrease in splanchnic circulation.

4. ANTIULCER DRUGS WITH GASTROPROTECTIVE ACTIVITY: ANTACIDS, CARBENOXOLON, SOLON, SUCRALFATE, AND COLLOIDAL BISMUTH

Soon after the discovery of the cytoprotective activity of PG, numerous studies were carried out to determine whether a similar activity might be attributed to classic antiulcer drugs, which were believed to act primarily by gastric acid inhibition. It was soon realized that a wide variety of such drugs exert cytoprotective-like effects. Anticholinergics and H_2-receptor antagonists, which are potent inhibitors of gastric acid secretion, offer rather mild protection, primarily against acute gastric damage induced by such ulcerogens whose damaging action is partly pH dependent (aspirin, cysteamine, taurocholate, or restraint–stress). These antiulcer drugs (except pirenzepine) may even augment ethanol-induced lesions, suggesting that their protective activity in other models of gastric injury could be partly related to their gastric inhibitory effects. Omeprazole was also reported to prevent acute gastric mucosal damage induced by ethanol, but this effect was only observed after oral administration, suggesting that it may be attributed to a mild irritant effect of omeprazole on the mucosa.

The prototype of gastroprotective drugs used in the ulcer treatment is carbenoxolone, synthesized from glycyrrhizic acid, a constituent of licorice. Pretreatment with carbenoxolone significantly reduced acute gastric mucosal lesions induced by various irritants. Carbenoxolone does not effect gastric acid secretion. Therefore, its gastroprotective and ulcer healing could not be attributed to the inhibition of acid secretion but to other actions, such as stimulation of mucosal PG and/or inhibition of LT, the decrease in pepsin secretion, the increase in mucus secretion, and the prolongation of the half-life of mucosal cells. Since the gastroprotection can be defined as the prevention of acute gastric damage by a mechanism other than the inhibition of gastric acid secretion, carbenoxolone could be considered as a typical gastroprotective drug.

Carbenoxolone is rarely used clinically because of some aldosterone-like side effects. Synthetic derivatives of sophoradin, an extract of ancient Chinese medical plant (*Sophora subprostata*), which has a profile of action similar to that of carbenoxolone, but no side effects, is now widely used for the treatment of gastric ulcers in Japan. This interesting drug, known as Solon, has been shown to protect rat gastric mucosa against a variety of ulcerogens, including ethanol, aspirin, restraint–stress, and bile salts. It is a potent stimulant of mucosal generation of PG and an inhibitor of LT and Tx formation, resulting in increased mucus–alkaline secretion, mucosal blood flow, and rapid mucosal cell restitution, following damage to the mucosa. Solon or similar compounds seem to have a therapeutic potential but further study is required to document its protective and antiulcer efficacy in humans.

Antacids containing aluminum hydroxide and magnesium hydroxide such as Maalox or Mylanta II are generally considered to act mainly as acid-neutralizers, but several recent reports suggest that these drugs exhibit gastroprotective effects that cannot be explained simply by reduction in gastric acidity. Tarnawski *et al.* reported that Mylanta II protected rat gastric mucosa against 100% ethanol in the rat. Szelenyi found similar protection by antacids against aspirin- and taurocholate-induced damage. Possible protective effects of antacids unrelated to reduction of luminal acidity include the binding of pepsin and bile acids, strengthening of the mucus–alkaline barrier, and stimulation of endogenous PG release. Antacids containing aluminum hydroxide enhance the healing of chronic peptic ulcerations at both lower and higher dosages, but it is unknown whether acid neutralization may be only one of the mechanisms by which these agents promote ulcer healing.

Sucralfate (basic aluminum salt of sucrose octasulfate) and De-Nol (colloidal bismuth subcitrate) have been long used in peptic ulcer therapy. Recently these agents became the subject of special interest because of their gastroprotective activity. These drugs are not antacids, since their acid-neutralizing capacity

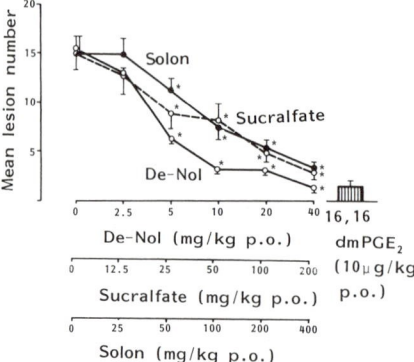

Figure 6. Mean lesion number in the rat stomach exposed to absolute ethanol without and with pretreatment (30 min before ethanol) using various doses of Solon, sucralfate, De-Nol, or 16,16 dmPGE$_2$. Mean ±SEM of 8–12 rats per dose of drugs used. Asterisk (*) indicates significant decrease below the control value obtained with ethanol alone.

is almost negligible, but they exhibit some antipeptic activity either by forming complexes with proteins, thereby depleting pepsin of its substrates (sucralfate), or by direct inactivation of pepsin by bismuth ion (De-Nol) by means of a chelation process. Both agents interact with the mucus gel by adhering to the mucosal surface, thereby effectively decreasing its permeability to acid and pepsin and thus reducing direct attack of luminal acid and pepsin on the mucosal cells. Both sucralfate and De-Nol bind EGF in a pH-dependent fashion. These drugs can increase the concentration of EGF in ulcerated areas by several-fold, possibly enhancing the healing activity of EGF. The antipeptic effects of both sucralfate and De-Nol prolong the half-life of EGF in the ulcerated areas perhaps increasing EGF's stimulating activity.

Sucralfate and De-Nol can prevent gastric mucosal lesions induced by a variety of ulcerogens, including absolute ethanol, bile salts, restraint–stress, aspirin, and indomethacin (Fig. 6). This wide range of the gastroprotective effects of sucralfate and De-Nol resembles that of PG. Hollander and Tarnawski were the first to demonstrate that the protective action of sucralfate is mediated (at least in part) via release of endogenous mucosal prostaglandins and that sucralfate interacts with the normal gastric mucosa increasing the defensive capabilities. Subsequently several studies have confirmed that sucralfate and De-Nol affect the mucosal production of PG. Indeed, we and others have found that both sucralfate and De-Nol increase the mucosal generation and luminal release of protective PG, such as PGE$_2$ and PGI$_2$, while reducing the tissue level of LTC$_4$ (Fig. 7). The mechanism of stimulation of PG formation by sucralfate and De-Nol is unknown, but it may be attributable to the activation of mucosal macrophages. PG mediation of the gastroprotective activity of sucralfate and De-Nol is only one part of their protective mechanisms since these drugs can also

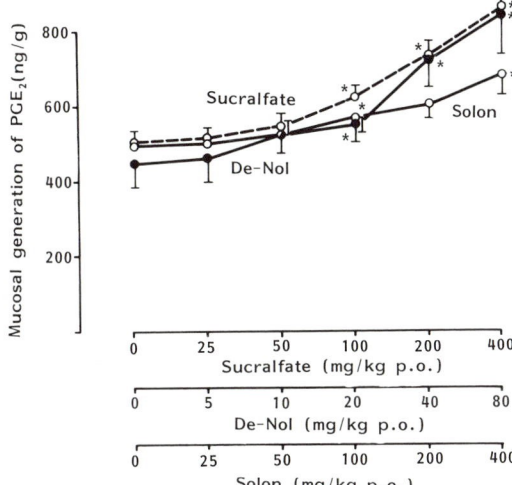

Figure 7. Mucosal generation of PGE$_2$ in rat fundic mucosa treated with various doses of Solon, sucralfate, or De-Nol. Mean ±SEM of 8–12 rats per dose of drugs used. Asterisk (*) indicates significant increase above the control value obtained with saline treatment.

prevent the mucosal damage induced by NSAID when the mucosal formation of PG is almost completely suppressed (Fig. 8).

Both sucralfate and De-Nol have been used to protect the gastric mucosa against aspirin damage in humans. The results showed clearly that the drugs were effective in the prevention of aspirin-induced gastric microbleeding and endoscopic erosion formation (Fig. 9). The mechanism of this prevention has yet to

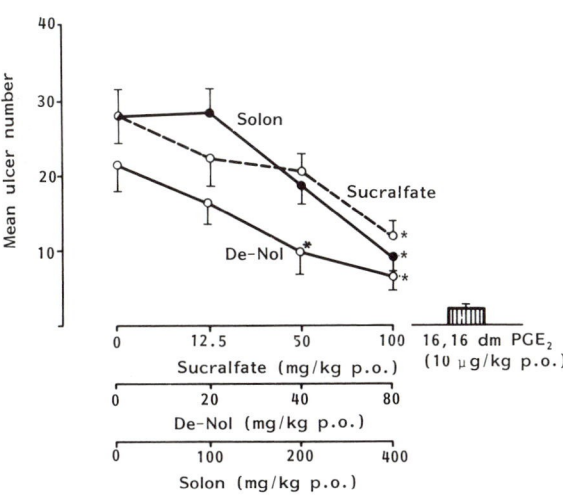

Figure 8. Mean ulcer number in the stomach exposed to acidified aspirin (ASA) (200 mg/g) in rats without and with pretreatment with various doses of Solon, sucralfate, De-Nol, or with 16,16 dmPGE$_2$. Mean ±SEM of 8–12 rats per dose of drugs used. Asterisk (*) indicates significant decrease below the control value obtained with ASA alone.

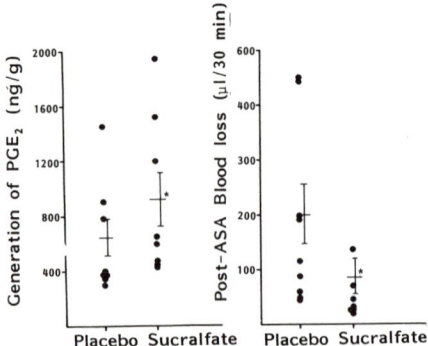

Figure 9. Effects of 4-day treatment with sucralfate (4 g/day) on gastric microbleeding and DNA loss (measured in gastric washings) induced by aspirin (2.5 g) in 8 subjects. Asterisk (*) indicates significant change as compared to the value obtained in tests with placebo.

be elucidated, but the strengthening of the mucus barrier and the reduction in mucosal LT generation may be major factors in their protective activities. Thus, the currently available results indicate some beneficial effects of sucralfate and De-Nol in the prevention of NSAID-induced gastric mucosal injury in humans.

Numerous well-controlled clinical studies have demonstrated that sucralfate and De-Nol significantly enhance the healing of both gastric and duodenal ulcers. Furthermore, these drugs appear to reduce the relapse rate of ulcers healed through their action. The possible contribution of gastroprotective effects to antiulcer efficacy and to the prolongation of ulcer remission by sucralfate or De-Nol require further investigation.

5. OTHER NONPROSTAGLANDIN GASTROPROTECTIVE SUBSTANCES: SULFHYDRYLS, MECIADANOL, CERTAIN INORGANIC COMPOUNDS, PAPAVERINE

Szabo *et al.* (1981) suggested that naturally occurring nonprotein sulfhydryls (SH) such as glutathione are important initiators of mucosal protection. Therefore, several SH-containing agents have been tested for possible gastroprotective activity. Among such SH agents, cysteamine, *N*-acetyl-L-cysteine, and dimercaprol were reported to partially protect the rat gastric mucosa against ethanol damage; by contrast, SH blockers, such as iodoacetamine, abolished PG-induced gastroprotection. The concept implicating SH in gastroprotection remains controversial, however, because unexpectedly, certain SH depleters, such as diethyl maleate (DEM), were found to exert cytoprotection.

Flavonoids are ubiquitous substances that may affect various steps of cyclo-oxygenase or lipoxygenase pathway. Meciadanol is a stable flavonoid without any acid-inhibitory or neutralizing effect, but it is highly effective in preventing the gross and histological damage induced by 100% ethanol, aspirin, or restraint–stress. It appears to be without any influence on the mucosal generation of PG but reduces histamine content because of the inhibition of histidine decarboxylase activity and reducing the tissue level of histamine. It is unknown whether this antihistamic effect could contribute to gastroprotection by Meciadanol.

Several inorganic compounds containing zinc, copper, selenium, tellurium, cadmium, chromium, and so forth, have been reported to provide some protection of the gastric mucosa against ethanol damage. Their mechanisms of action are under investigation, but the scavenging of oxygen free radicals or the increasing of tissue SH have been proposed.

The intragastric administration of papaverine was found to inhibit significantly gross and histologic gastric mucosal damage produced by 100% ethanol. Papaverine is a potent inhibitor of smooth muscle contractile activity; it also appears to stimulate the mucosal production of PG. It is likely that this drug, used in humans mainly for its smooth muscle relaxant effects, could be useful in mucosal protection by PG-mediated mechanism.

6. CONCLUDING REMARKS

From this review, it is obvious that a wide variety of drugs exert a gastroprotective effect against different types of experimental gastric mucosal injury in animals and humans. The list of gastroprotective substances is rapidly growing. H_2-blockers or anticholinergics offer little protection (limited to pH-dependent mucosal injury). Other agents, including antacids, carbenoxolone, Solon, sucralfate, or De-Nol, are effective in a variety of experimental models of gastric damage and resemble the protective efficacy of PG. Whether the increase in mucosal generation of PG or the reduction in LT play any role in the protection has yet to be determined. These protective drugs may be recommended to prevent mucosal injury in patients receiving NSAID and other irritants. Most other cytoprotective agents, that either suppress the generation of damaging products of cyclo-oxygenase (Tx2) and lipoxygenase pathway (LT), or stimulate mucosal growth (gastrin, EGF), or act by some unknown mechanism are purely experimental compounds awaiting future clinical trials to examine their possible clinical value in preventing or healing gastric mucosal damage in humans.

ANNOTATED BIBLIOGRAPHY

Braquet P, Etienne A, Mencia-Muerta J-M, et al: The role of platelet activating factor in gastrointestinal ulcerations. *Eur J. Pharmacol* 1988.
  Study indicating that PAF may contribute to gastric damage in endotoxine shock and restraint stress and that PAF antagonists prevent PAF- and endotoxin-induced mucosal damage.

Gregory H: Isolation and structure of urogastrone and its relationship to epidermal growth factor. *Nature (Lond)* **257**:325–328, 1975.
  Early review describing the structure, origin, and biological action of EGF and urogastrone.

Guth PH: Mucosal coating agents and other nonantisecretory agents. Are they cytoprotective? *Dig Dis Sci* **32**:647–654, 1987.
  Recent review of gastroprotective drugs and substances and their mechanisms of action.

Hollander D, Tarnawski A, Gergely H, Zipser RD: Sucralfate protection of the gastric mucosa against ethanol-induced injury: A prostaglandin mediated process? *Scan. J. Gastroenterol.* **19**(Suppl 101):97–102, 1984.
  First demonstration that protective action of sucralfate is dependent (at least in part) on release of endogenous mucosal prostaglandins.

Hollander D, Tarnawski A: Protection against alcohol-induced gastric mucosal injury by aluminum-containing compounds—sucralfate, antacids and aluminum sulfate. *Scand J. Gastroenterol.* **21**(Suppl 125):165–169, 1986.
  Paper discussing the role of aluminum-containing compounds in protection of the gastric mucosa against injury.

Konturek SJ: Gastroprotection by antisecretory and non-antisecretory agents. *Klin Wochenschr* **64**:24–27, 1986.
  Review of gastroprotection induced by agents inhibiting and noninhibiting gastric acid secretion.

Konturek SJ: Role of epidermal growth factor in gastroprotection and ulcer healing. *Scand J Gastroenterol* **23**:249–254, 1988.
  Review article on the involvement of EGF in gastroprotection and ulcer healing.

Konturek SJ, Brzozowski T, Drozdowicz D, et al: Role of leukotrienes in acute gastric lesions induced by ethanol, taurocholate, aspirin, platelet-activating factor and stress in rats. *Dig Dis Sci* **33**:806–813, 1988.
  Study showing deleterious effects of LTC4 and PAF on the gastric mucosa and their prevention by LTC4 receptor antagonists.

Konturek SJ, Brzozowski T, Piastucki I, et al: Role of prostaglandin and thromboxane biosynthesis in gastric necrosis produced by taurocholate and ethanol. *Dig Dis Sci* **28**:154–160, 1983.
  Study showing that gastric mucosa generates Tx and that Specific Tx synthesis inhibitor (OKY 1581) prevent taurocholate-induced mucosal damage.

Konturek SJ, Brzozowski T, Radecki T et al: Cytoprotective effects of gastrointestinal hormones, in Miyoshi A (ed): Gut Peptides and hormones, Tokyo, Biomed Res Found 1982, p. 411.

Konturek SJ, Dembinski A, Warzecha Z et al: Role of epidermal growth factor in healing of chronic gastroduodenal ulcers in rats. *Gastroenterology* **94:**1300–1307, 1988.

Study showing that endogenous EGF secreted by salivary and duodenal glands plays an important role in healing of chronic gastroduodenal ulcers via stimulating mucosal growth.

Konturek SJ, Kitler ME, Brzozowski T, et al: Gastric protection by meciadanol. A new synthetic flavonoid-inhibiting histidine decarboxylase. *Dig Dis Sci* **31:**847–852, 1986.

This paper provides an evidence that the inhibition of histamine formation by suppressing histidine decarboxylase activity in gastric mucosa prevents acute gastric lesions induced by ethanol or aspirin.

Konturek SJ, Pawlik W: Physiology and pharmacology of prostaglandins. *Dig Dis Sci* **31**(suppl):6S–19S, 1986.

Review of physiological role and pharmacological effects of prostaglandins.

Konturek SJ, Radecki T, Brzozowski T, et al: Antiulcer and gastroprotective effects of Solon, a synthetic flavonoid derivative of sophoradin. Role of endogenous prostaglandins. *Eur J Pharmacol* **125:**185–192, 1986.

Study on the gastroprotection induced by Solon and its mechanisms.

Konturek SJ, Radecki T, Brzozowski T, et al: Gastric cytoprotection by epidermal growth factor. Role of endogenous prostaglandins and DNA synthesis. *Gastroenterology* **81:**438–443, 1981.

First study showing that EGF protects gastric mucosa against aspirin damage via PG-independent mechanism.

Konturek SJ, Radecki T, Piastucki I, et al: Gastroprotection by colloidal bismuth subcitrate (De-Nol) and sucralfate. Role of endogenous prostaglandins. *Gut* **28:**201–205, 1987.

Study showing that both De-Nol and Sucralfate prevent the formation of acute gastric lesions induced by various irritants and that it may be attributable, at least in part, to an increase in the mucosal generation of PGs.

Kusterer K, Rohr G, Schwedes V: Gastric mucosal protection by somatostatin. *Klin Wochenschr* **64** (suppl VII):97–99, 1986.

Study showing that somatostatin protects the gastric mucosa against various irritants.

Lacy ER, Itoh S: Microscopic analysis of ethanol damage to rat gastric mucosa after treatment with a prostaglandin. *Gastroenterology* **83:**619–625, 1982.

Study showing that prostaglandins do not prevent the destruction of surface epithelial cells by absolute ethanol, questioning the concept of the cytoprotection.

Olsen PS, Poulsen SS, Kirkegaard P, et al: Role of submandibular saliva and epidermal growth factor in gastric cytoprotection. *Gastroenterology* **87:**103–108, 1984.

Study demonstrating gastroprotective effect of endogenous and exogenous EGF against cysteamine-induced mucosal injury.

Peskar BM, Lange K, Hoppe U, et al: Ethanol stimulates formation of leukotriene C4 in rat gastric mucosa. *Prostaglandins* **31:**283–293, 1986.

Study showing deleterious effect of LTC4 generated in ethanol-treated gastric mucosa and possible prevention of this damage by LT inhibitors.

Robert A: Cytoprotection by prostaglandins. *Gastroenterology* **77:**761–767, 1979.

Proposition of the concept of direct cytoprotection induced by exogenous PG and adaptive cytoprotection by mild irritants acting via releasing endogenous PG.

Robert A, Nezamis JE, Lancaster C, et al: Cytoprotection by prostaglandins in rats: prevention of gastric necrosis produced by alcohol, HCl, NaOH, hypertonic NaCl and thermal injury. *Gastroenterology* **83**:619–625, 1982.

First study showing macroscopic prevention by prostaglandins of acute gastric mucosal damage by various necrotizing substances.

Silen W: Gastric mucosal defense and repair, in Johnson LR (ed): *Physiology of the Gastrointestinal Tract*, ed. 2. New York, Raven, 1987, p. 1055.

Review chapter on the mucosal defense mechanism against various noxious agents, emphasizing the importance of rapid restitution of mucosal cells in the recovery of the mucosa from the damage.

Szabo S, Trier JS, Frankel PW: Sulfhydryl compounds may mediate gastric cytoprotection. *Science* **214**:200–202, 1981.

Study showing that endogenous and exogenous sulfhydryl compounds may be initiators of gastroprotection.

Takeuchi K, Johnson LR: Effect of cell proliferation and loss on aspirin-induced gastric damage in the rat. *Am J Physiol* **243**:G643–G468, 1982.

Study indicating that gastrin may contribute to the gastroprotection against aspirin-induced mucosal damage by a mechanism involving stimulation of mucosal growth and epithelium proliferation.

Takeuchi K, Johnson LR: Pentagastrin protects against stress ulcerations in rats. *Gastroenterology* **76**:327–324, 1979.

First study demonstrating that pentagastrin protects against stress ulceration, possibly through stimulation of growth of gastric mucosa.

Tarnawski A, Hollander D, Gergely H, Stachura J: Comparison of antacid, sucralfate, cimetidine and ranitidine in protection of the gastric mucosa against ethanol injury. *Am. J. Med.* **79**(2C):19–23, 1985.

Study demonstrating that sucralfate and antacid protect the gastric mucosa against alcohol injury while H_2 blockers, cimetidine and ranitidine not only do not offer protection but in fact may increase alcohol-induced damage.

Tarnawski A, Hollander D, Krause WJ, Stachura J, Gergely H: Does sucralfate affect the normal gastric mucosa? Histologic, ultrastructural and functional assessment in the rat. *Gastroenterology* **90**:893–906, 1986.

Experimental study demonstrating interaction of sucralfate with normal gastric mucosa in rats in a manner increasing its defensive capabilities.

Tarnawski A, Hollander D, Stachura J, Mach T, Bogdal J: Effect of sucralfate on the normal human gastric mucosa. Endoscopic, histologic and ultrastructural assessment. *Scand. J. Gastroenterol.* **22**(suppl 127):111–123, 1987.

First endoscopic, histologic and ultrastructural study demonstrating interaction of sucralfate with normal human gastric mucosa.

Wallace JL, Whittle BJR: Profile of gastrointestinal damage induced by platelet activating factor. *Prostaglandins* **32**:137–141, 1986.

Study describing the deleterious effects of PAF on the gastrointestinal mucosa.

Whittle BJR, Vane JR: Prostanoids as regulators of gastrointestinal function, in Johnson LR (ed): *Physiology of the Gastrointestinal Tract*, ed 2. New York, Raven, 1987, p. 143.

Extensive review of endogenous arachidonate products involved in gastric damage (Tx, LT) and protection (PG).

Index